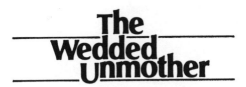

The Wedded Unmother

KAYE HALVERSON
WITH KAREN M. HESS

AUGSBURG Publishing House • Minneapolis

To all who struggle with crisis

Contents

Introduction   9

1   As American as Mother and Apple Pie   12

2   First Comes Love, Then Comes Marriage   22

3   Time to Start Our Family   32

4   If At First You Don't Succeed . . .   45

5   Valleys, Valleys, and Then Some   60

6   Coping   84

7   Resolution   100

Epilog   119

Resources   122

Introduction

Should I read this book?

YES, if you are trying to become pregnant and are possibly infertile. This book depicts my struggle in dealing with infertility—alone, unable to find any help in understanding the pain I was feeling because of infertility. Alone—or so I thought. Yet 10 million of us experience infertility at one time or another in our country. One out of six couples of childbearing age are involuntarily childless. We are not alone.

YES, if you are a parent or relative of someone who doesn't have children. You may have concluded they don't want to have a family, but, in reality, they may be dealing with infertility, learning to cope with the various stages of this crisis.

YES, if you are a friend of someone struggling with infertility. It is often difficult to relate to others if you haven't been through what they are experiencing. You may have children already. Your friend may envy you, making it difficult for her to relate openly and honestly. Be understanding and patient.

YES, if you wish to rid yourself of stereotypes implanted in us by previous generations, namely: (1) when you grow up you'll get married, and (2) you'll start to raise a family shortly thereafter.

YES, if you are interested in how one struggles with faith in God when dealing with crisis.

A book which relates to your personal needs can become an understanding friend. That is my greatest hope for this book—that it will be an understanding friend to many, in doctors' offices, in ob-gyn clinics, in infertility clinics, in hospital lounges, in adoption agencies, and, most of all, in the homes of those who feel deep pain because of infertility. I can talk about it now, and I hope that this book, written out of the depths of the pain of dealing with infertility, will help you to understand, deal with, and talk about infertility too.

I was determined to share our story in the hopes of helping others. Yet writing this book became part of my therapy too, one of my ways to resolve our infertility. God does, indeed, work in mysterious ways. So often when we set out to help others, we help ourselves as well.

A special thanks to my husband, Craig, for his enduring love and patience during my identity struggle and my personal life crisis—infertility. Thanks also to my parents and family, who encouraged me to write this book, especially to my father, who saw to it that I made a serious effort to get it published. Finally, thanks to Augsburg Publishing House for giving me this opportunity to share our story with others and for introducing me to the remarkable and most compatible Dr. Karen Hess, who has been a special joy to work with.

Kaye Halverson

1

As American as Mother and Apple Pie

Sometimes we wait too long before we get around to questioning our assumptions.
—Nathaniel Branden

It was a crisp, cool Minnesota day of my junior year at Gustavus College. Social gatherings, fall "rush" activities, and class assignments filled my world. At the moment, class assignments were top priority. I had to write a paper for a religion class on the topic "Religion and Where I Am Now."

An easy assignment. I knew where I was and what I wanted out of life, and I assumed I had complete control over my future. My own energy, ambition, and faith in the power of God left little to chance. I had come a long way in my first 20 years of life, and religion had played a large part. My father is a Lutheran pastor. From my earliest years I attended church school, church camp, and church functions regularly. I vividly recall attending weddings and baptisms and imagining Father performing *my* wedding ceremony and baptizing *my* children—his grandchildren.

When I was in elementary school, being a minister's daughter brought a certain prestige, perhaps due to the times—early 1950s—or to living in a small, rural community in Minnesota. I always felt important and special as the minister's daughter. I had few worries as a child. My girl friends and I spent hours playing house. I was always a happy wife with two adorable little girls and one handsome little boy.

We were a close family, working together, playing together, and, above all, talking together. My mother was a 5'6" blue-eyed blonde whose sensitivity, compassion, and organizational abilities made her the perfect minister's wife—or so I assumed. And my father—I assumed he was the perfect minister. Tall and dark, with brown eyes and a warm, friendly smile, he was tireless and completely dedicated to his work, perhaps over-dedicated. He would spend 80 to 90 hours a week counseling those who were ill, lonely, depressed, bereaved, or divorced. The Monday Funeral Syndrome spoiled many of our planned family outings. Monday was supposed to be Dad's day off, but month after month, because of the unpredictability of death, funerals were scheduled on Monday. Consequently, Father seldom had a day off. For therapy he would come home and knead Mother's bread dough, and we would talk about next Monday and the things we might do together.

We moved during my sixth year of school, and being

the new girl in town gave me a certain status, for about a month. After that I was the Preacher's Kid—P.K. How I hated that label! I imagined people could tell from my very appearance that I was a P.K. I attributed the typical frustrations, anxieties, and uncertainties experienced by all adolescents to my unique P.K. status. At times my self-consciousness was almost unbearable. My face would flush and my heart would pound while doing something as routine as walking down the church aisle to the front pews with my mother and sisters.

My parents never forced me to participate in high school church activities. It was just expected that I would, and I did. I was also expected to encourage my friends to become members of the High League and the church choir, a role I often resented. As I experienced the typical teenage peer pressure, my rebellious spirit started to surface. Participating in religious activities became more of an obligation to my parents than an experience I totally enjoyed. Although my parents never gave me the feeling I *had* to belong, I felt it was something I ought to want to do.

I began to question church doctrines, and one summer during my sophomore year in high school I informed my parents I wanted to attend some other churches. To my surprise, they encouraged me. It was then I realized that even if my father had not been a minister, I would have been brought up in much the same way. My parents raised me according to what they truly felt and believed, not just according to what was right for a P.K.

Christ never tested me personally through my high

school years, except maybe through my middle sister, Mary. Mary was born with minimal brain damage with an emotional overlay, a condition for which there were no medical guidelines, no known case histories to study. She had my mother's blonde hair and blue eyes and a fabulous memory for trivia, yet she was unpredictable. She envied the popular kids in school and tried hard to be part of their clique. Her growing pains and ours could be a story in itself, as we all were tested emotionally in seeking happiness for Mary. We prayed together that she would be happy and mentally healthy.

My sister Ruth was five years younger than I, a "kid," and now that I was in college, we were not especially close. I knew little of her present world other than that she was a musical mini-star and got very good grades. I assumed once we both finished school, got married, and had children, we would regain the closeness we had shared in our younger years. I was looking forward to being "Aunt Kaye" to her children.

My parents worked hard to send me to a private Christian college. My mother worked part-time to help with my expenses and with Mary's staggering medical and special teaching expenses. I worked too, every summer from eighth grade on.

Now, with two years of college behind me, I was quickly becoming an authority on everything, especially religion. My weekly religious metamorphosis depended on what lectures I attended that week and what new theories and philosophies I wanted to try. One night I called home and chatted incessantly, not really listening to what my parents had to say. Mother remembers my last comment being: "By the way, I don't believe in God any more. See you next weekend."

The wonders of being a college authority! However, my parents weren't greatly concerned about my flippant comment. They, too, had been college students. Knowing of my great enthusiasm for new experiences in life, they found my comments almost humorous.

The following weekend I went home, anticipating a long talk with Mom and Dad, eager to tell them about all that had happened since the start of the term. But that weekend it was my turn to listen. Involved in my fun-filled, challenging college world, I had assumed that all was going smoothly at home. I had no idea that a power struggle in the church had been emotionally and spiritually draining my parents. Two or three influential church board members had decided that it was not suitable for their minister's wife to teach school. Neither was it suitable for their minister to give piano and voice lessons or to play the organ at the country school and in the newly organized summer theater on his day off. They even criticized my parents for attending movies. These men viewed any activities of their minister and his wife which were outside the church as being "unorthodox." My father felt it might be best to leave this parish.

My first reaction to the news was disbelief. How could Christians cause another devoted Christian to give up his home and his life's work simply because he had far-ranging interests and did not devote every waking hour to religion? My disbelief turned to anger and then to outright rage. I made an appointment with

16

one of the pillars of the church and let him know in no uncertain terms that I didn't need this kind of Christianity.

I was dating Craig Halverson at the time, one of my high school sweethearts and now my college "love." Craig was 6'2", a brawny business major who liked hunting and fishing. He played football, baseball, and tennis in high school and college. Craig knew our family well. In fact, one summer he drove my mother and Mary down to Oklahoma to a private school, an emotionally and physically draining experience. Craig also knew of my frustrations with the church. He helped us try to understand the few church members who were causing the crisis in our family.

Dad finally decided that, although the majority of the parish wanted him to remain, he could not continue with political tensions and confrontations distracting him from his mission as a minister. My parents moved east to a new synod. The experience did little to build my faith in organized religion.

In the coming months, I realized more and more my mother's spiritual strength as she sought to free Dad of his depression and to find suitable living arrangements for Mary and a new job for herself. Her belief in God as the only source of power to get her through life day by day never wavered. I wondered if my faith would be as strong, should I ever be tested so severely.

I returned to college and was again quickly wrapped up in studies and sorority-fraternity activities. One evening Craig and I were out on a country road "parking." With Craig's strong arms around me, I felt the conflicting emotions of peacefulness and security and excitement and frustration. I wondered often what it would be like to really make love rather than only kissing and cuddling, but I would wait to find out until I was married. Fortunately, Craig shared this conviction.

I had a strict curfew at Gustavus, and soon it was time for me to return to campus. Craig started the car— and the wheels spun in the mud. Stuck! I was dismayed. We'd never get unstuck in time! My fears were unfounded, however. Craig, always prepared, had an old rug, sand, and a shovel in the trunk. In no time we were out and on our way. I thought to myself, "Now here's a fellow who would make a terrific husband and father."

Craig and I were engaged in the spring of my junior year. We planned to be married the following year. I remember sitting in my classes writing possible names for our children:

Heidi Marie Halverson
Chad Weston
Halverson
Sara Anne
Halverson

I assumed that after we married we would surely have a family. Why did I make this assumption? Were billboards, commercials, movies, television shows, and Mother's Day cards subconsciously ingrained into my plans for the future? I don't know where this assumption came from. "Tradition," I guess, as in *Fiddler on the Roof.*

Why was I going to marry Craig? I loved him, at least as far as I knew about love at that time. But above all else, he would be a terrific husband and father.

We often double-dated with Lanna and Rick, also high school sweethearts, who were planning to be married the same summer as we. Lanna and I talked and fantasized about our marriages—how we would handle unfaithful husbands, how many children we'd have, what color schemes we'd use in our homes. I dreamed about Sunday afternoons of wedded bliss. I'd be stretched out on the couch, smelling my apple pie baking in the kitchen and watching Craig play with our little ones. The contented wife and mother.

At one point I was nervous about marrying Craig because I didn't think he talked enough. My friends and their boyfriends talked for hours on the phone. Craig would just call up, ask for a date, and that was it. His letters didn't compare to those Robert Browning and my fantasy man wrote. But we had a lot of fun together, and that was important too.

I was also somewhat concerned about my premarital exam, but I needn't have been. My doctor was very knowledgeable about family planning, presenting various alternatives. For Craig and me the Pill seemed the best choice. The doctor advised that we plan to have our children before we were 30. "Of course, we'll want children as soon as we get ourselves situated," I responded.

I went out East the holiday before graduation, completely engrossed in wedding plans and student teaching. Our family was invited to a Christmas gathering at a delightful couple's home. The hospitality and Swedish glögg were superb. We spent the evening singing Christmas carols and playing silly games.

After we left, I asked my mother how all these people were related and which ones were the children of our host and hostess.

"They don't have any children," replied my mother.

"No children? Why not?"

"I guess perhaps they couldn't have any."

"Why not?"

"Not everybody can have children, you know."

No, I didn't know, or at least I had never thought about it. This was my first conscious recognition of childless couples, and I wondered why I had never been aware of them before.

"Well, why didn't they adopt a child?" I asked.

"Adoption isn't always for everyone either."

"Why not? Didn't they *want* to have children?"

"There are no children for some."

Mother's response left me speechless.

Stereotypes, assumptions—where do they come from? My parents gave me a wide variety of growing experiences. They did not raise me to believe that my sole purpose in life was to get married and produce children. Yet I assumed my role in life was to be a wife and mother.

Now I had more important things to consider than other people's infertility. I was getting married on June

24. I would teach elementary school in Edina for two years, and then we'd start our family—two or maybe even three children. We'd see how it went with the first two. After all, we didn't have to decide that today.

2

First Comes Love, Then Comes Marriage

Whither thou goest, I will go;
and where thou lodgest, I will lodge:
thy people shall be my people,
and thy God my God.

—Ruth 1:16 KJV

Our honeymoon, spent on Mackinac Island, Michigan, was flawless, but much too short. In no time we were headed back to establish our home together. Throughout the drive I wished I had some cookbooks along to read. I had done next to nothing in the kitchen and was apprehensive about how I would keep Craig as happy as his mother, an excellent cook, had done for the last 21 years. Craig also enjoyed cooking, so I was naturally nervous about my inadequacies.

The first task facing me when we reached our apartment was to make a grocery list. Like Mother Hubbard's, all our cupboards were bare. I pored through cookbooks, planning complete menus for each meal as meticulously as I prepared my teaching plans. Leftovers never entered my mind; each meal would be a masterpiece, or so I hoped. My shopping list grew longer and longer. Since we didn't even have salt, flour, or sugar, each recipe added 10 to 15 items to the list. Ironically, by the time I finished the list and Craig and I completed the shopping, no time remained to fix the delight I had planned for our first dinner. We dined at McDonald's.

Once our kitchen was fully stocked, however, cooking became an interesting challenge. We were never quite certain how any meal would turn out because we continuously experimented. I was becoming more confident in my culinary skills and decided to try a special spicy fruit dessert called Hurry Fruit Curry. It was so hot we threw the entire dish down the disposal. I felt like a failure, but not for long. My next creation was scrumptious.

Our love of experimenting with cooking carried over to our entertaining. We delighted in creating special hors d'oeuvres that looked and tasted exotic, yet fit our budget. The media had some influence on the image we were trying to create. As I prepared for an evening of entertaining, flashes of television commercials depicting an elegant hostess gracefully balancing a silver tray of delectable pastries would remind me that I should polish the silver tray we'd received as a wedding gift. I never did get around to it though; there just was never enough time.

The media influenced our sex life also. We were indoctrinated on the wonders of the Pill during the sexual revolution in the early '60s. We would not leave having children up to chance, nor would we risk contributing to the world population problem. We would plan carefully. I was sure that if I took the Pill and then quit, I would become pregnant. So, like most of my friends, I took the Pill. Craig and I both had jobs and we were saving for a house. We felt a house was far better than an apartment for raising children, so, it was only wise to wait to start our family. Typical. Very typical.

Our first year of marriage dispelled my earlier fears that Craig might be difficult to communicate with. Whenever I needed to talk, he was always ready, not only to listen, but to talk with me. We prayed together before going to bed, always closing with, "I love you." Falling asleep nestled in Craig's strong, protective arms filled me with joy and contentment. Marriage was all I had hoped for, and more.

After two months of being the "perfect housewife," I started my first year of teaching fourth grade. It was a fun year with many new experiences, new friends, new responsibilities, and a new dog. Peppi, an adorable little ragmop, soon became an important part of the family.

Our limited budget never crimped our social lives. We had our first Christmas party in our apartment, and since paper dresses were in vogue that season, I bought a floor-length Hallmark Holly dress for the occasion. I worked so hard on last-minute preparations that I perspired holes through the underarms. "I'll just keep my arms down, and no one will notice," I thought, forgetting my natural impulse to hug people I care for. But holey underarms soon became secondary.

We were sitting around singing Christmas carols when Peppi, still all puppy, bounded into the room and greeted each guest. She had already become quite a little show-off. Finally, to impress everyone with her newest accomplishment, she trotted over to me and proudly proved that she was paper trained—on my new dress. Merry Christmas!

The remainder of the school year flew by, and, in what seemed like only a few months, we had been married an entire year. On our first anniversary we decided to start an anniversary tradition of listing the high points we'd shared the past year. We had a lot: small trips, good friends, good jobs, our church, our families, and most important, each other.

We started toying with the idea of my going off the Pill, but then we were also thinking of buying our first house. Soon we did just that—a three-bedroom split-level with a huge backyard as dry and sandy as the Big Sahara, as we fondly called it. We agreed to pay back the money we borrowed for the down payment in three years. We could wait three more years before having children. Perhaps I could go off the Pill in two years and we'd just "chance it" the last year.

Occasionally I'd forget my Pill. Then I'd be nervous and edgy until I got my period. One month, shortly before Easter, I had forgotten to take a Pill right in the middle of my cycle, and my period was a week late. Certain I was pregnant, Craig bought a little stuffed chicken for the baby that Easter. But I wasn't pregnant, and we were both tremendously relieved. We saved the little chicken for future reference.

Wedded bliss continued. We were settled into a comfortable routine when, the week before fall workshop was to start, Craig came home and announced that we had a chance to go to Los Angeles for six to eight months. Although we had only been in our new home for two months and I was starting to teach in a new school district, we were always ready for new experiences. We rented our house, packed some bare essentials, and were off to California in our '67 Mustang.

We stopped at Gustavus to see my sister Ruth before heading west. I baked a specially decorated cake for her and felt very motherly, since our parents were now settled in Buffalo, New York. Ruth, too, would be more alone without family so close. We cried our good-byes, but they were mainly tears of happiness, as we both loved our lives.

The drive to California was breathtaking, especially the Rockies. Oray, Colorado, seemed to us a lot like what Switzerland must be like. We ate at a little restaurant called the 6/24, our anniversary date, so we asked the waitress if we could have a plate to keep. She readily agreed. Fond memories.

In "beautiful downtown Burbank" we found a pink and turquoise apartment with a central tropical garden and pool which we thought was smashing. Craig worked for Sperry-Univac on a Lockheed Aircraft special project. I was free to come and go, to shop, to sit by the pool, and to eat, and eat, and eat. I put on 25 pounds for my record high of 155. I also did some sewing, my biggest project being a striking red wool pantsuit with a cape that I planned to wear when we returned to Minnesota. We both let our hair grow and I felt we were emerging into new personalities. I started putting dark brown rinses in my hair, imagining I was becoming more ravishing with each rinse.

We had a chance to return to Minnesota earlier than expected. After spending money for four solid months, eating almost all our meals out, and taking side trips here and there, we were ready to get back to our home, friends, and family, especially since Christmas was almost upon us. We had experienced the "good life" and were ready for the better life—the comforts of a real home. Also, thoughts of starting our own family were becoming more frequent. As the time drew nearer, it became harder and harder to postpone.

We arrived in Minnesota with only two days to move back into our house, decorate, and prepare food for Christmas. However, our anticipation and enthusiasm were so great, it seemed effortless. With snow falling and Christmas carols playing on the stereo, we prepared for one of the best Christmases ever. We finished rushing around just before Craig's parents arrived. Again, my parents were not able to be with us, but the excitement of celebrating Christmas in our own home helped fill that void. The greatest treat was seeing Craig's mom and dad again. His dad had just retired and was looking forward to having time to relax and enjoy hunting, fishing, and coin collecting. We told them all about our California days. We took many pictures, including a special photo of Craig and his dad playing cribbage.

Life was, indeed, full and good to us. Craig's brother

and his family joined us for Christmas Eve church services. I gave special thanks to God for the safe trip home and for being together as a family and starting a new episode of life.

The next week we were invited to ML and Rick's apartment for a welcome-back holiday party. I wore my new red pantsuit and cape, and my rinsed hair was long, dark brown. Unfortunately, my "smashing" home-made outfit did nothing to help create a new me, because the added 25 pounds was splitting out the pants' zipper. As for my newly tinted hair, pictures from that Christmas tell me it was not as ravishing as I had imagined.

It was a memorable evening back with old college friends. During the evening we young women got around to talking about our marriages and our plans for the future. We talked about how great it was not to have to worry about children right now, to be free to do what we wanted. We all planned to have children; we all assumed we would. The only questions were when and how many. Craig and I left the party feeling fortunate to have such good friends and such a good life.

Our happiness was shattered in two short weeks, however, when Craig's father died from a heart attack. We were stunned. For both of us, this was the first loss of a close loved one. I had just started teaching sixth grade, so I took a week off to be with Craig and his mother. We were so thankful for that last Christmas together. We realized more than ever before how important family was to us. We talked about how good

"Grandpa" had been to his grandchildren, and we wished our children would have had a chance to know and love him, and he them.

Perhaps it was Craig's father's death, or perhaps it was Craig's gentle yet persistent comments that I was being too hard on the church and that I should forgive and forget. Whatever the reason, we became more active in our church as choir members and High League advisors. Being a "yes" person, I was soon chairing several committees and heavily involved in a variety of activities, work-related as well as social.

Since I grew up in a home where religious discourse thrived, I joined churchwomen's groups and tried to become involved in their Bible studies, but I found them to be quite cold. Most of the women were used to doing things the way they had always been done. I was convinced that, with a little creativity, the group could be warmer and more responsive. The night it was my turn to be Bible lesson leader, I suggested we all sit on the floor to be more comfortable and close, and that we hold hands for the opening prayer. The hostess stated flatly, "We're all comfortable right where we are."

Perhaps I was too idealistic, but again I had strong misgivings about some aspects of organized religion. I was certainly not stimulated by these sessions. Other aspects of the church, however, compensated for this loss.

Through our church we became close friends with two other High League advisors, Diane and Bob. Diane was a kindergarten teacher who shared my interests in sewing and education. Bob was a fun-loving sixth-grade teacher and assistant principal. He liked working with wood and doing home projects, and he shared Craig's interests in sports. They lived only a few blocks from us, so we got together often.

When it was time for my yearly pap smear and checkup and to renew my Pill prescription, a friend recommended a gynecologist downtown. I didn't mind the 10-mile drive downtown to his office just this once, but I figured when I got pregnant I would find a gynecologist nearby. We hoped it wouldn't be much longer before we would be parents and give our parents grandchildren.

Our parents didn't prod us to start a family. Since mine were so far away, our summer get-togethers at the lake were always a series of long catching-up sessions. The subject of children came up frequently, and they knew that children were a part of our plans.

We were able to get together with Craig's mother more often. Being naturally chatty, I enjoyed standing in the kitchen wiping dishes with her and expounding on my philosophy of child-raising. Since we were both elementary teachers, we shared many ideas on the "real root" of children's difficulties. Although we often held opposite philosophical views, we usually agreed on practical matters.

One weekend when we were visiting Craig's mom, one of her friends dropped by and, upon seeing me petting our dog, queried, "Won't it be more fun to take such good care of a baby? Haven't you started thinking about a family yet? You surely will be good parents now that you've got all that running around out of your systems."

Comments such as these became more frequent after our second anniversary. It was like a magic turning point in life. Suddenly we were expected to start a family. Still, when someone asked, "Do you have any children?" it was not difficult to respond, "No, not yet." Not too long, in the almost near future, we would have our one and then our two.

The next Christmas we drove to Buffalo with Craig's mom and my sister Ruth to spend a week with my parents. It was our first Christmas with them since we'd been married. We had a fabulous time caroling in the snow and sharing long hours of conversation.

Being young, in love, and married meant many special moments and new experiences with new friends. Soon we would share more new experiences with a newborn child in our family. I started decorating the third small bedroom in our home in pink, a good color for a sewing room. Of course, it wouldn't remain a sewing room for long. We put our aquarium in the room so no one would think we were too obvious. To most people a small, pastel room means only one thing: a baby.

It would still be a while before we learned. There are no children for some.

3

Time to
Start Our Family

Who knows most, says least.
—Alexander Pope

Our planning had worked out perfectly. I was not
pregnant yet and our home loan was almost paid off.
We had been lucky. We were secure in our jobs. I
thoroughly enjoyed teaching sixth grade and had many
positive experiences with the children and other teachers. Our home was adequately furnished, our material
needs met. We enjoyed our lives to the fullest and were
satisfied in our expectations. We had been married more
than three years. Now we were eager to start our
family.

I went off the Pill. I was certain I would be a "fertile
Myrtle," like some of our friends who went off the
Pill and immediately became pregnant. We didn't mind,
however, when I didn't get pregnant the first few
months because that meant I could finish out the school

year and we could keep to our three-year plan for paying back our home loan.

We weren't concerned with how quickly I would conceive. We had much to occupy our time. We never announced that we were starting our family, and neither did any of our friends. They only announced when they had something real to announce: pregnancy. And more and more of our friends were making announcements.

One evening I was playing bridge with my good friend Sandy when the conversation turned to the population problem. Sandy matter-of-factly stated, "Andy and I decided when we first got married that we wouldn't have children."

"You're kidding!" I responded. "Why not?"

"We just felt that the world is so overpopulated, in such a sad state of affairs, that we didn't want to bring children into it."

"You'll probably change your mind sometime."

"No, I don't think so. Have you read Paul Erlich's *Population Bomb*?"

"No, I haven't, but I'm planning to."

"Dr. Erlich encourages having no more than two children per family, or better yet, none. When you read it, you'll see why we feel so strongly about our decision."

Sandy was not unique in her feelings, but the decision to be child*free* surprised me. Many of our friends were now pregnant, and baby showers were becoming more and more frequent. I gave a number of showers for good friends, each time feeling a deep sense of admiration as I noticed the change in their bodies, the special feminine look they acquired for which I deeply longed. Even their maternity clothes looked special And their husbands were all so proud and loving. I was becoming very impatient for *our* turn.

That winter we took a ski trip to Lutsen with some friends, two of whom were pregnant. There was lots of talk about gas pains and heartburn and comparisons as to whose was worse. I was quite unsympathetic toward the discomforts of pregnancy; certainly they were worth putting up with to have a child. However, as the week progressed, I grew more self-conscious when the conversation turned to pregnancy and I had nothing to contribute.

One evening as we were gathered around the fire in the lodge after a long day of skiing, the talk turned to children's names, possible delivery dates, and what sex the children would be. I recalled the statement of Dr. James A. Peterson in *Toward a Successful Marriage:* "The ideal image of marriage in America seems to include the crib and the baby buggy." I promised myself I was going to reread that book after we got back from our ski trip. Was Dr. Peterson promoting the stereotypes which were now hurting me and making me feel inadequate?

The first chance I got after we returned home, I took out *Toward a Successful Marriage* and began reading. Chapter Eight, "The Infant in the Family," contained the statement which I had recalled with anger at the lodge. The chapter implied that couples can and should choose when the blessed event of childbirth will take place and that 85% of all marriages result in children. This was followed by a paragraph on infertility and how it has increased from 5% 75 years ago to 15% today:

A woman reaches her highest peak of fertility in her mid-twenties and if her initial pregnancy is delayed too long after that she may not succeed in having a baby. Besides their pattern of living should not become so fixed that it is difficult for them to adjust to an infant.

I closed the book, upset. I was supposed to be at my peak fertility, yet I was not pregnant.

The following summer some friends invited us and a few other couples for a weekend at their parents' cabin. We took our new black toy-miniature poodle, Tasha, with us. We seldom left her home; she had become our "baby," as is typical of many young couples with no children. The weather was perfect, and it was great renewing old friendships. Surprisingly, none of us had children yet, and we all had our dogs along. We took "family portraits" of each couple and their dog, laughing as we attempted to find family resemblances between parents and children. My friend's father commented, "You'll all surely be good parents. Look at how you adore your dogs."

Her mother laughingly joined in, "When are you going to start thinking about Pampers instead of doggie treats?"

We were! And we wondered how many of our friends were too. Craig and I talked about it all the way home. It really was no one's business but our own, yet the subject kept coming up, putting us on the defensive.

One evening our friends Lanna and Rick told us they were planning to adopt a child because they probably were not going to be able to have a biological child. (You will never hear me say "one of their own," which implies that adopted children are not really the adoptive parents' own children.) Although Lanna and Rick had briefly mentioned their infertility problems, we were surprised that they were taking steps to adopt so soon. They had been going to an infertility clinic, but were making no headway and had been told that perhaps they would only have children by adopting them. They were worried that the ease of adoption might change. Rick had accepted a four-year position in Germany beginning the next year, and they hoped to adopt a child before they left the country.

Luck was with them. They received Shawna Beth three months before they left. Shawna was a beautiful child: lots of dark hair, big blue eyes, a creamy complexion—a living Dresden doll. We were thrilled when Lanna and Rick asked us to be Shawna's godparents. The whole idea of adoption seemed very natural and acceptable because they were so comfortable with their decision.

Holding Shawna, feeling the closeness of an infant, and seeing Rick and Lanna's happiness, I became even more eager for us to have a child too. I'd been off the Pill for over a year now. I became extremely depressed each month when I got my period. Being naturally impatient, I made an appointment with a second gynecologist to see if he could speed things up.

The waiting room was filled with pregnant women. I pretended that I, too, was pregnant but not showing yet. How fun it would be to flaunt my fat tummy when we finally succeeded.

The nurse's call, "Kaye Halverson," interrupted my fantasy, and I followed the nurse down the hall and into an examining room. After a brief wait, the doctor entered, and we had a lengthy discussion about pregnancy. He examined me, advised me to start taking my basal body temperature (BBT), and asked me to check back in four to six months.

Some of my close friends now had their first babies. Their happiness, the showers, those cuddly new babies were so exhilarating, I could hardly wait a day longer for *our* turn. I visualized our little boy as built just like Craig, and I wondered if I would let him go off hunting with his father when he was a toddler or if I'd insist that he wait until he was older. Our little girl would have big brown eyes like me and would be a real companion.

Lanna and Rick were so pleased with their adoption that they encouraged us to register with the same agency. They had only waited for Shawna one year, but their social worker told them the adoption scene was changing rapidly. We thanked them for their concern and advice and then wished them bon voyage.

After their departure, we began to spend more time with Diane and Bob, our High League advisor friends, who were also considering adoption. We discussed the topic often, and finally the four of us went to Lanna and Rick's agency and filled out applications. We were told that the waiting period for a Caucasian infant could easily be six to seven years. Craig and I were amazed, but not troubled. We would probably have a biological child by then and could adopt a second child. We might even want to adopt a child of another race. Diane and Bob, however, were upset at the long waiting period and unhappy with their social worker. They applied to another agency.

One Sunday at church a neighbor stopped to comment on the darling dresses of two little girls. Then she asked, "Kaye, when are you going to start your family?" It was the first time I had been asked the question so directly, and I was speechless. Unable to respond to her question, I murmured, "Yes . . . adorable."

Lanna and Rick asked us to come visit them in Germany. We decided to use our savings and go to Europe that summer. We planned all spring, eagerly anticipating the trip. I couldn't help but recall hearing that a relaxing trip away from one's normal routine, a change of pace, was ideal therapy for couples trying to have a baby. I continuously calculated how many more months of teaching I'd have if I was pregnant next month. Just enough time left to save for this . . . and that. . . .

We left in June for our three-week trip, and it was worth every penny. We visited France, Italy, Germany, the Netherlands—a fun-packed three weeks. We were delighted with Shawna Beth and how she had grown, as well as with what good parents Rick and Lanna seemed to be. I told Lanna I was frustrated about not being pregnant yet, but we didn't spend much time discussing it because, in my heart, I refused to believe I was infertile.

Still not pregnant after our European trip, I compensated by immersing myself in activities. Some friends and I created a Christmas craft club and made homemade goodies for the coming holidays. I took guitar lessons, a graduate course in education, and an upholstering course, redoing a chair in velvet for our living room. Time sped past.

Craig and I were still enjoying being High League advisors. Craig also played broomball and hockey and went ice fishing in the winter. He and a friend bought a fish house and put it out on what we called the Dead Sea, because take-home catches were nonexistent.

We spent Christmas Eve alone—by choice. Some of the joy of Christmas was gone; we still had no child to hang a stocking for. Determined not to let our childless status spoil Christmas, I agreed with Craig that we spend Christmas Day with his family.

The following summer I took my crafts to various local art fairs, an interesting, enjoyable diversion. I began to think seriously of changing my vocation, perhaps doing greeting card illustrations and messages.

We continued to receive birth announcements and shower invitations. Would our turn *ever* come? I started to paint Pennsylvania Dutch symbols and created one of the distelfink for our home. The theme was fertility, good luck, and good fortune. Although I was not superstitious, I figured it couldn't hurt.

My sister Ruth was planning to be married, and she and Jack decided on a Christmas wedding. Our home would be the base for the wedding and reception. It was an especially exciting time of year, combining Christmas and wedding festivities. We had a small party for Ruth and Jack in our home, with champagne and all the trimmings. All was fun and merriment until one of my parents' friends asked me directly about our family plans. I responded, "Yes, we are interested in having a family, and we have also placed our name with an adoption agency." I had been forced to make a statement about our childlessness, and I felt extremely uncomfortable. Later Craig and I discussed the need to handle these comments together, but he was rarely asked such questions, so it became more my problem than his, especially since I was the one who reacted so negatively.

After the festivities of the wedding and Christmas, the weather turned bitter cold. I felt depressed, utterly discouraged. I made another appointment with my gynecologist. He recommended a series of tests. I was put under sedation, so I couldn't drive home from the clinic myself. One of Craig's friends drove him to the clinic to get me. I was concerned that his friend might wonder what I was having done and that others might know how hard we were "trying" to have a baby.

We left town that night for a weekend visit with Craig's mother and decided not to talk about the medical tests. As was typical, during dishwashing after meals, Craig's mother and I chatted about school and work, and I philosophized on how we were going to raise our family. Our parents still didn't pressure us to have children, but we knew they would be extremely happy when we did.

Our niece stayed overnight one weekend shortly after that. She and I did artsy-craftsy things together, enjoying each other's company greatly. I was taken aback, however, when she stated that when she was married and had kids, I would be a grandma. All I could think to respond was, "We can't always tell what our future holds."

I tend to overreact when people flatly state that they are going to start their family, and I find it difficult to believe that it happens that easily for some. I know it does, but I feel strongly that those who grow up with that assumption have the hardest time adjusting to the contrary. When friends say they'll probably start their family next year, I have the strongest urge to say, "Don't assume anything; one never knows."

Craig says, "Forget it. Most people have the right to assume this will be true." But must we encourage that assumption? Perhaps along with the marriage certificate should come a little gold-embossed card bearing the words of Albert Ellis: "The commonest assumption among married people is that they should have children. The next most common assumption seems to be that children increase the happiness of a given marriage. There is little evidence to support these assumptions."

Yet most people want and strive to have children. I was strongly impressed when I read that Mo Dean, wife of Watergate's John Dean, said they were going to Europe to rest and then would start their family. I had a great curiosity about people my age and older without children. Were they like me? Had they suffered? Would they ever need someone to talk to? Or had they chosen not to have children?

I also wondered how older people with young children handled that adjustment. I saw a picture of my college's new president and family. The parents looked at least 40, and they had two small, darling children. I was excited to read that the woman had interests similar to mine. It made me feel I was OK, that there was still hope for my future and that of our children.

That fall a friend confided that she had just had an abortion. She was concerned about my reaction because she knew we wanted to have children and that we also had strong religious convictions. I assured her I believed each couple had to make their own decisions, and I was sure theirs had not been an easy one. Still, I couldn't help but question God's design in allowing her to become pregnant when she did not want a child and refusing Craig and me this gift.

A few weeks later I hosted our monthly bridge club. As usual, the conversation got around to children before we had completed the first rubber. Erica got us all thinking when she said, "Have you ever asked yourself, 'Why do I want kids?' Maybe we want to have someone to love us back. Is that selfish?"

"Or so we won't be alone on the holidays? Christmas . . . what will we do at Christmas?" added Sandy.

Nodding concurrence, Karen said, "I must admit, honestly, that I want children so I can have some

42

cuddling and loving. My husband isn't that way. We love each other a lot, but he wasn't raised to show affection openly. My family did, and I crave that loving and hugging."

"Try a puppy," chided Jan.

That hit a nerve, and I heard myself asking, "Are we nuts over our pets because we don't have kids?" Seven responses merged into a blur: "Of course not." "Maybe so." "Who knows?" "What!" "Impossible." "Very possible."

One Sunday shortly after that conversation, I was deeply moved by the scripture verse in the church bulletin. I cut it out and taped it to our refrigerator:

May God who gives patience, steadiness, and encouragement help you to live in complete harmony with each other—each with the attitude of Christ toward the other. And then all of us can praise the Lord together with one voice, giving glory to God, the Father of our Lord Jesus Christ (Rom. 15:5-6 LB).

Patience was never one of my attributes. I'd had little need for it. My life had worked out quite the way I had chosen—until now. In reading this passage, I prayed that I would not be jealous of my friends who had children or were becoming pregnant.

Why couldn't I feel like Sandy did? Sandy and her husband chose not to have children. Still very conscious of the population problem, they had decided the child-free life was not for them and had opened their home to foster children. "I feel we're doing our part to help out the world," Sandy would say, "by not having a family. And then we think we are helping by taking in foster children."

"Don't you ever get outside pressure to have children biologically?" I once asked.

"No, we made our position very clear to friends and relatives in the beginning," was her simple answer.

But I wasn't as noble as Sandy. I wanted to have a family, and yet I was beginning to wonder if it might be true for Kaye and Craig Halverson that . . . there are no children for some.

4

If At First
You Don't Succeed . . .

One ship drives East, and another West
While the self-same breezes blow
'Tis the set of the sail and not the gale
That bids them where they go.

Like the winds of life are the ways of Fate
As we journey along through life.
'Tis the set of the soul that decides the goal
And not the storm or the strife.
— Ella Wheeler Wilcox

Although many of my friends were starting to have their families, I didn't consider myself a rare specimen yet. However, I decided it would be wise to investigate more fully, to have an "infertility work-up."

During my first visits, the doctor checked my reproductive organs and asked about Craig's and my sexual habits. He went over my BBT charts I'd kept for a year and asked personal and nonpersonal questions about childhood diseases, family diseases, and my background. "Do you know how to have babies? How often do you try? Do you enjoy it?" He said that the male can be equally responsible for an infertility problem. The next step would be having Craig examined.

Craig and I had both heard parents make statements such as "They had to adopt because *he* had some difficulty." That's what *her* parents would say. *His* parents would say they had to adopt because *she* couldn't get pregnant. Someone was always at fault. We promised each other we would never place blame if we continued to have problems; the outcome would never affect our love. We also agreed not to discuss it with anyone. This was personal, nobody else's business.

Secretly, though, I believed the tests would show that Craig had the problem. I was preparing myself to help him with this adjustment, to give him special love and encouragement — as if he needed it, my stable, well-adjusted husband.

The first test meant getting a sample of sperm to the laboratory for analysis. It sounded very simple, but it wasn't. The laboratory was 20 miles away, and the sperm had to be delivered fresh. We were always trying to deliver a specimen when we had to get to work or it had just snowed or the car wouldn't start or there was a traffic jam.

Additionally, there was some embarrassment delivering the specimen. Craig never complained about doing this, for which I was very grateful. He jokingly said it was much less embarrassing than his first trip to the clinic when he arrived empty-handed, unaware that he was to have brought a specimen along. "That's embarrassment," he grinned.

Craig's sperm count was found to be low, so he was put on medication—very expensive medication—and the count rose. Soon he was diagnosed as being all right. Our hopes soared. A problem had been found and corrected.

We also learned of and tried to control many other factors which can affect conception: having a good breakfast, drinking little alcohol, not smoking, controlling weight, taking warm rather than hot showers, and Craig wearing shorts rather than briefs. We tried everything, becoming more and more impatient.

Our sexual relations became extremely frustrating. Having sex for its own sake was impossible, because timing became essential. Conflict arose between sexual desires and rational desires to conceive a child. I felt a growing sense of personal inadequacy and a whole gamut of other negative feelings relating to infertility.

By now most of our friends—fat ones, drinkers, smokers, breakfast-skippers, brief-wearers—were having their babies. Appointments with the gynecologist, four to six months apart, were too infrequent to satisfy me. After two years of seriously trying to conceive, and with so many friends now pregnant, the question "Do you have children?" elicited a terse *no*. I felt even tenser trying to verbalize an acceptable answer to the oft-accompanying question, "When do you plan to start having your family?" I fought valiantly to keep my thoughts, feelings, and frustrations hidden and

47

refused to let "outsiders" know of our struggles. By now I was convinced it was *my* problem, a situation I was not at all prepared for.

It was even difficult for me to talk about children. My feelings changed often. One month I desperately wanted to get pregnant, and the next month I talked myself into not caring if it happened this year or next. Then I'd read or hear more about Zero Population and other new theories, and I'd grab on to one of them for a month or so. Our friends began to avoid the topic. I'm sure they thought I was super-sensitive—and I was.

What I really needed was a chance to discuss the problem frequently. Fortunately, I had Craig, a great husband with two enormously large ears and one tremendous-sized heart full of love and empathy. Yet he personally felt that whatever happens, happens, and we do what we can. He didn't seem to care how our family situation turned out because he believed we had a very good life already. I was glad to know that deep down he was quite happy with just me. Yet his attitude also left me feeling that I was carrying the burden alone.

I did have a close friend from whom I never had to hide my true feelings. She understood totally how one day I could say I didn't want children and how the next day I was dying to be a mother. Gradually, I began to communicate with others too. I learned that several friends were having similar problems, so I didn't feel quite so alone.

On my next visit my gynecologist discovered that I might have endometriosis, a disease of the uterine lining. He suggested I go to an infertility clinic specializing in this area. A close friend of mine had also been suggesting that I try the clinic. One of her friends had gone there and had soon become pregnant.

Although I thought it was a good idea, I kept putting off making an appointment, perhaps not wanting to exhaust what might be my last chance at solving our problem. Since I was teaching, it was hard to make a private phone call, and by the time I got home, the appointment desk was closed. However, I finally got around to calling, naively believing that I could get an appointment for the next week. What a joke! It took almost a day to get the correct office and number. Then the only woman who made appointments for the doctor's new patients was out for the day. When I finally reached her, she said she would send me an application form to complete. It arrived a full week later. I immediately completed it and mailed it back. A month passed before she called to arrange my first appointment—for four months later! I was disappointed, depressed—but not defeated, not yet.

The four months dragged by, but the big day finally arrived. I took time off from school and eagerly headed for the clinic. I had been married six years, trying to get pregnant for three years, and waiting for an appointment for four months. This was finally it. All my questions would be answered, all my problems solved. God was waiting for me inside that office door; he would help me.

After hassling with parking and getting my bearings, I was slightly ruffled when I arrived. There were forms, forms, forms to complete, and then the wait. I'm seldom bothered by waiting for appointments. I always take a bag of time-fillers with me: papers to correct, letters to write, magazines to read—time-fillers galore. Nevertheless, after two hours, I began to get impatient. I asked at the desk how much longer and was told that the doctor spends a lot of time with his patients and not to worry, I'd be called.

After another two hours, I was so frustrated, depressed, and irritated that I was sure it was noticeable. The silence in the waiting room was stifling and uncomfortable.

Finally I was called, taken to an inner room, and told to undress. I sat for another half-hour before a resident entered, got some information, and left. I sat for another hour. Just as I was about to get dressed and find out what was causing the delay, a nurse came in to tell me the doctor had been called to the hospital for an emergency; I'd have to come back another day.

I couldn't believe it. I was hysterical inside, but controlled myself until I got to my car. Then I cried and cried and cried. As I left the parking ramp, I told the attendant I'd pay the first hour, but they could send the rest of the *#+#*! bill to the clinic. The flabbergasted attendant offered no rebuttal.

Three months later I got my next appointment. I again took the day off from school and again hassled with traffic and parking. And, as before, I sat more than two hours in the waiting room. Finally I went to the desk and asked if there was a problem. Unfortunately there was. They had lost my chart, and the doctor would not see a patient without a chart. I told the nurse in no uncertain terms that I was not going home again because they had lost my records; they had bloody well find them or I'd have a nervous breakdown right in front of them. The records were quickly "found," and I was soon ushered in. I was an emotional wreck by that time and imagined I also looked like a physical wreck, but at last I was about to meet the great doctor. I soon found that he was as good as his reputation.

He first reviewed with me the general procedure in an infertility work-up and gave me an information sheet to share with Craig. He explained that the principal cause of infertility is attributed to the male in approximately 39% of the cases, to the female or to combined causes in 60%, and to the technique of intercourse in only 1%. "Must be due to 99% of the couples having read *The Joy of Sex*," I thought to myself. He explained that an estimated 15% of the population experiences infertility at one time or another and that this is a fluid statistic because a couple is classified as experiencing infertility if they have not conceived after one year.

After the doctor reviewed my previous files and tests, he scheduled me for a laparoscopy and a possible laparotomy, during which a scope would be inserted through my navel to check out my insides.

I was excited about going to the hospital, optimistic that something would be discovered and our problem solved. However, I had also heard stories about hospital patients being mixed up and undergoing the wrong type of surgery, so I was apprehensive. I was prepared to take a month off from work because it was possible I would have a fairly long recuperation, depending on what occurred during surgery. I scheduled a good substitute for my class and hoped the children would miss me while I was away and not enjoy the substitute too much.

It was a week before Thanksgiving, an ideal time to have a few extra weeks off. On the way to the hospital, I jokingly told Craig to stay with me all the time before surgery or they might mistake me for a heart patient and wheel me in for open-heart surgery. Ironically, we arrived to find the hospital so crowded that they had no room for me in the ob-gyn ward, and I was given a room in the heart ward next to a heart patient in a coma—not very pleasant surroundings, especially in view of my lighthearted comment to Craig less than half an hour before. I truly worried that they might actually mistake me for a heart patient and whisk me off for surgery on the wrong end.

My parents, who had moved to Atlanta, called that evening to see how I was doing. I knew my mother desperately wanted me to say, "Please come and be with me," and she would have flown up immediately. But since they were planning to come for Christmas, I felt they shouldn't spend the money. I assured her that I would be just fine. Later I wished I had encouraged her to come. The experience proved much more difficult than I imagined.

I was glad to see Craig bright and early the next morning before they wheeled me into surgery. He assured me they had me scheduled for the right procedure and not to worry, he'd be close by.

I was in surgery for more than five hours, and even Craig was getting concerned. The doctors found extensive endometriosis, a buildup of tissue in the uterine lining that makes it extremely difficult to get pregnant. The disease may cause scarring and ovarian adhesions or cysts and is often accompanied by painful periods or even painful intercourse.

I awoke the next morning, groggy, and saw tubes in the veins in my arms. I was shocked and terribly afraid that something horrible had happened during surgery. Of course, I was being fed intravenously, but I was not prepared for that. The tubes were taken out as soon as I came to. Then I reached down and felt the stitches, the "bikini incision," as they called it. I would be staying in the hospital for a week.

It was painful to walk, but I had to exercise a little every day. Although I was next to the maternity ward, I didn't go see the babies until two friends came to visit and insisted on going. We laughed at the cute babies and the homely babies, but inside I was being torn apart.

The day I was to go home, the doctor told me to start taking the Pill again to keep the endometriosis from growing and to create a state of false pregnancy, thereby enhancing my chances of getting pregnant when I went off the Pill—in nine months! I was to take as many as needed to control the bleeding and discomfort, and keep him posted on how I was doing.

I cried all the way home. Would I ever leave the

hospital cuddling our long-waited-for child? I wished I could talk with my grandmother, whom I had called from the hospital. Although she stayed in a nursing home several miles away, she and I were very close. Perhaps she could help me understand why I kept crying uncontrollably.

Almost as if by fate, a letter from her was waiting for me when we arrived home. I recognized the handwriting, firm and strong for a woman in her mid-80s. Eagerly, I opened the letter and read:

Dear Kaye and Craig,

It was good to hear your voice. So like Romans 8:28, "All things work together for good." I know, Kaye, how anxious you both are to have a child, but cheer up; it can happen to you yet. [She told how many of her relatives waited several years for their children and how some adopted children. They all went through periods of anxiety, yet everything turned out well for them.]

I believe God can work miracles even in this day according to *his* will, and we know, too, that our prayers are answered, sometimes no, since his way is best. Faith is ceasing to worry, leaving the future to God, who controls the future.

Keep looking up, keep happy as you are, and keep a happy home. You are a special teacher and serving the Lord in a special way. I am sure the children love you. A good teacher has a mission to mold young lives.

Love,
Grandma

I felt warm and close to her and loved her for taking time to write to cheer me up and for coming straight to the point of my primary concern. So often people avoid discussing anything controversial or painful. I greatly appreciated the warmth of her letter, and it had come at just the right time. I reread it, folded it carefully, and placed it in the little box containing my other treasured mementos.

Ruth and Jack came down from Duluth to share Thanksgiving with us. Ruth took care of everything, bringing the turkey and all the trimmings. Being a nurse, she took good care of me. Craig, also an outstanding "nurse," enjoyed being in charge of making me feel chipper.

I began to look forward to Christmas and, since I had the month off, I started making Christmas decorations by building a giant gingerbread cookie house. It was great fun.

We had another wonderful Christmas with our families. My mother was very concerned about my surgery and asked a lot of questions, but it was difficult for me to discuss it. Although I wanted to talk about it, my feelings were confused. I always had great hope we would have a family—whether biologically or through adoption—but neither seemed very probable right now.

Diane and I became closer following my surgery. We both were feeling sexually and personally inadequate because of the possibility of infertility, and we both were eagerly waiting for news about our adoption applications. We often talked about who would get her child first and how the other would react.

Diane was not pursuing medical help because her husband was diabetic and they felt adoption was the wisest option. They were content with that decision. We often discussed adoption, its ramifications, and the difficulties of parenting an adopted child.

Since most adoption agencies see themselves as the advocate of the child, we had to be our own advocates. Although we tried not to let the social workers at the agency intimidate us, we tended to tread lightly when discussing our concerns with them. Since they were screening us, to offend them might mean we would not be given a child.

We had both read the text of a lecture on adoption services given by David and Ruth Kirk ("The Challenge of Change") and agreed wholeheartedly with their statements:

In the period before a child is placed with them, adoptive applicants are likely to experience very strong feelings, typically of deprivation, anxiety, sorrow, over-sensitivity, frustration, and perhaps of personal inadequacy. In women, these feelings are likely to be strongly felt and overtly expressed. Men typically express themselves less forcefully, and a good many say they are concerned only because of their wives' feelings. There are a number of things adoptive applicants can be taught that are likely to enable them to make the best use of these feelings.

Diane and I were bolstered by Kirk and Kirk's observation that infertile couples make excellent parents for adopted children:

Infertile adopters must be taught that facing their own pain over their infertility and/or childlessness will make them better able to feel with, to have empathy with their adopted child. Having learned to face their pain and deal constructively with it, and remembering what it is like to FEEL pain, they can better understand their child's pain over being re- linquished, and his need to understand.

We were both very concerned about the long waiting period and the drastic change in the adoption scene. I read in Victoria Salkman's *There Is a Child for You* (Simon and Schuster) that, until 1969, 75% of all children born out of wedlock were placed for adoption; only 25% were kept. In contrast, today 92% are kept by the biological mother. Salkman states that more and more people want to adopt, but that healthy white in- fants are at a premium because of (1) contraception and abortion; (2) unwedded mothers keeping babies; and (3) more couples, not only the infertile, wanting to adopt. Salkman also notes that persons wishing to adopt no longer have to be unable to conceive a child of their own, to be young, or to be married.

We talked about the lengths to which some people go to get a child. They use deception in filling out forms, apply to several agencies, or even buy a baby through the black market (sale for profit) or the gray market (sale for expenses). I saw a TV movie in which young, good-looking girls and boys were paid to con- ceive children for wealthy, childless couples and won- dered if this could actually be happening. Perhaps for some, the longing for children makes any means of satisfying this need acceptable.

We talked about what kind of child we might adopt: one just like us, one of a different background economi- cally, racially, or religiously; an infant, toddler, or school-age child. And we talked about how many children we'd like to adopt and how soon. If the opportunity to adopt more than one child at a time should arise, would we want this option? What if twins or triplets or an entire family of orphaned children were made available to us?

Another concern Diane and I shared was the current controversy over access to adoption agencies' sealed files and the rights of biological versus adoptive parents. What if we adopted a child and then the biological parent appeared on the scene and wanted the child back? What if our adopted child began searching for his or her biological parents later in life? We had much to consider.

In my search for answers, I began reading my Bible more diligently. A passage in Romans helped me:

If you are a teacher, do a good job of teaching. If you are a preacher, see to it that your sermons are strong and helpful. If God has given you money, be generous by helping others with it. If God has given you administrative ability and put you in charge of the work of others, take the responsibility seriously. Those who offer comfort to the sorrowing should do so with Christian cheer (Rom. 12:7-8 LB).

When I read this passage I felt my life had purpose—teaching and helping those in sorrow. I became involved in our church's Meals on Wheels program. I also fed a woman who had multiple sclerosis. She was very discontented, and it was difficult trying to cheer her up, but her troubles always made my problems seem minimal.

I often called my social worker at the adoption agency to see how things were progressing. After hanging up the phone, I would calculate how many more years of waiting remained. In only four years I would be past 30—a crucial point in the life of a prospective parent. Yet no one at our agency seemed empathetic concerning our infertility. No one ever said, "This must be very difficult for you, waiting so long for a child." I was never offered information on infertility or how to cope with the frustrations of waiting.

After being disappointed many times by phone conversations, I went to the agency to find someone to talk with or some material I could read. As I waited in the reception room to talk with our social worker, I looked at the list of dozens of pamphlets available. Titles included "Alone and Having a Baby," "Trans-Racial Parenting Groups," "Planning for Your Baby—An Adoptive Home." Every topic was covered *except* infertility.

Yes, I began to use the word. I was infertile. We were an infertile couple. Infertile and childless. A lonesome place to be. We were a completely neglected "species." A gnawing fear gripped me. Would we remain forever childless?

5

Valleys, Valleys, and Then Some

Is it so, O Christ in heaven,
that the highest suffer most,
that the strongest wander furthest,
and more hopelessly are lost?
—Sarah Williams, *In Twilight Hours*

The Pill again, and no hope of getting pregnant for at least nine months—how depressing. I had never known such misery. I blamed my depression on the Pill, and then became even more depressed at the thought of enduring such suffering for nine months. I cried uncontrollably at almost anything: a pregnant woman walking down the street, a friend announcing her pregnancy. Baby showers became impossible for me to attend. I felt pitied, atypical, and extremely vulnerable.

Commercials made motherhood extremely glamorous. Mother's Day and holidays, formerly happy family times, became difficult. Birthdays just made me feel older, without any progress toward set goals. Magazine articles were either geared at parenting or homemaking. Although I loved being a homemaker, I felt unsuccessful because we had no children. I pictured myself a failure, an inadequate, unfulfilled woman. I began to dislike teaching and became irritable with the children. Now I was a failure at my job, too. I lost all confidence in myself and went in and out of deep depressions. I coped publicly, but privately I fell apart.

Still, I had to go through the medical treatment if I hoped to get pregnant, so we stuck it out. How Craig lived with me during the next months, I'll never know. He ignored his own problems, concentrating on me and my needs.

I could no longer deny to myself that I was infertile, but I dreaded anyone else finding out, so I isolated myself from friends and even from family. I am naturally open, vocal, and honest, so it was difficult to keep my problems and concerns to myself, but I learned to role-play to hide my very personal, private grief from those I cared for.

Showers, baby announcements, and hospital calls on friends who had just had babies were continual now. Friends were having their second children, and I began to totally withdraw from their joy and excitement. I acted indifferently to their child-related joys and concerns and even cancelled out of a baby shower for a dear friend. Although I felt guilty, I simply couldn't cope with the shower festivities and the questions and comments I would inevitably receive about when I'd be having children.

I forced myself to think more of my career and started seeking out new friends who were childless. One such friend, Mary, was a teacher and a member of our monthly bridge club. She was older than I, and I wasn't sure if they were childless by choice, but she did mention they had applied for adoption at the same agency we had only nine months earlier.

One day Mary and I got into a lengthy phone conversation about our agency and its policies. She wanted me to join her in protesting the agency's policy on who was eligible for an adopted child. She felt that children shouldn't be placed with couples who already had children when the shortage was so apparent and the waiting list so long. We agreed that it should be one to a couple. However, I felt it would do no good to protest, and I didn't want a confrontation with the agency for fear they would think me a troublemaker and complainer and never place a child with us. Mary was disappointed in my lack of support, but she understood my position.

The next week, however, a conversation with a neighbor changed my mind. She was complaining about her children, one adopted and one biological, saying that her happiest days were when she was working and childless. Nonetheless, they were waiting to adopt a third child from our agency so their oldest child would have someone to talk to about adoption! Anger and hostility welled up inside me. How could the agency even consider placing a third child with her, or didn't they know her attitude? I couldn't understand placing a second or third child with families, especially families which didn't seem to appreciate them, when childless couples were waiting.

I phoned the agency and asked them directly about this policy. The response was, "We do not wish to play God by making decisions as to who should have children and who shouldn't." That made no sense to me. Weren't they playing God when they made the policy that there cannot be an age difference greater than 35 years between the parents and the child being placed? Craig was already 30, and I soon would be. With the tight adoption scene, we had to face the possibility that we wouldn't get our child before we were 35.

My social worker explained that biological mothers now had more control over the type of family their children would be placed with. The common prerequisites were: handy father, artistic and musical mother, good providers, other children in the family, living in the country or the city (depending on where the biological mother was from), and, unbelievably to me, *reborn* Christians. Reborn! It was now not good enough that we had been Christians all our lives. *Reborn* was better. I was bitter, hostile, and angry at the agency for honoring such requests.

I began to feel anger toward God also. Never in my life had I been angry with God. How could I be? God was loving and just, or so I'd been brought up to believe. But one morning as I was scanning the paper I came across an article about a pregnant woman in jail. What would happen to her child as she served a life sentence? I let out a bloodcurdling scream as I read. Craig came running from the shower and asked, "What on earth happened?"

I read the article to him, but it didn't upset him in the least. He simply put his arms around me, gave me a hug, and kissed me gently.

Why was I so upset? How could God see fit to give a child to a woman in prison, someone who could not even mother the child, when here I sat, ready and waiting for a child? I had prayed and prayed to God to give us a child. Communion on Sundays brought tears to my eyes as I knelt at the Lord's table asking for a child. Was I not praying correctly?

I became even harder on the church, asking more questions, searching for meaning, wanting ways to pray harder or more meaningfully. A number of fundamentalist friends offered me advice on what *true* Christianity should be: "If you really have faith, lay it in the hands of the Lord." "Read your Bible daily." "Pray correctly." I tried and tried, but I couldn't find peace.

I kept giving God chances to show me what I was to do with my life, but I was utterly frustrated in trying to let God show me the way. One friend told me to put a deadline on God and say, "I need to know what to do by midnight tonight, so let the telephone ring as a sign that my decision is right." Such clear, vivid signs never came my way, or maybe I was sound asleep by midnight. I never seriously believed I could give God an ultimatum. But I did need answers desperately.

I wished my parents lived nearer so we could discuss my misgivings about religion. My dad would surely help me put things back into their proper perspective, but this subject was not for writing about. Besides, I hated to write letters and never seemed to have time to get it all down on paper. I thought about calling to talk about my problem, but pride prevented it. They always said how proud they were of my independence and my ability to handle any situation. I couldn't let them know how badly I was floundering. So I isolated myself even from those I loved best.

I did share some of the medical aspects of my problem with Ruth, since she was a nurse and could understand and explain to me what effects the Pill was having on me. By now I was up to four Pills a day, and they were taking their toll physically and emotionally. I gained almost 15 pounds. That in itself was extremely depressing.

Was it the effects of the medication, or was my personality really changing? I could detach myself—stand to one side, watch my actions—and see that I was becoming a different person. So could Craig. I could be completely happy, walking home from some event, and upon seeing any parent-child interaction, become overtly angry and hostile—often toward Craig. Who else could I take my aggressions out on? And then I'd worry that I might lose him if I kept acting so terribly.

Craig was facing the same problem, but he was much stronger than I. His prime concern was *me*, my attitudes, feelings, and reactions to all the medication. He tried to prepare me for possible continued infertility after I went off the Pill by saying, "Kaye, you cannot fail at that over which you have no control." As far as

Craig was concerned, we didn't even have to pursue the medical route. He fully accepted the idea of adoption with a calm, cool detachment, insisting that the outcome didn't matter. He was emotionally prepared for whatever our "fate" might be. Although I kept insisting he must have stronger feelings on the subject, they never surfaced, so it became *my* crisis.

I called our adoption agency again, asking for someone to talk with about infertility, but they said they couldn't help me. "Why not?" I asked. "There must be others like us, experiencing infertility and waiting for adoption." The answer was cool and calculated: "We don't want someone to handle that unless they are fully qualified. It's a very emotional situation." As if I didn't know! Still, they would not give me the name of anyone in a situation similar to mine.

I tried to put the matter out of my mind by involvement in nonchild-related activities. When it was my turn to host the antique club, I prepared for it with a happiness I hadn't felt in months. Talk would center on antiques, not babies and diapers. However, as the women browsed around my home, I overheard comments such as, "You surely can tell that Kaye doesn't have children. Why, she'd never have all these lovely things around if she did," and "She could never keep her house this clean and spotless if she had kids running around." I felt tears well up, a lump in my throat, and a deep, painful longing for a child's mess in my home.

I forced myself through the meeting, hoping no one would notice my red eyes or my silence. So many assumptions and stereotypes of this type about childless couples need to be chiseled away. We so often hurt others deeply with quick impressions and assumptions about their lives.

Rather than being stereotyped by our friends, why can't we receive love and understanding? Often when I was with some of my closest friends, I wished they would open the subject of our family planning. I couldn't just come out and say, "Guess what? We're going to adopt a child in four or five years." But no one asked. Silence. Isolation.

I really wanted to talk about being childless and alternatives to the situation and began searching for others who shared the problem. I found another friend, Sarah, who had quit teaching to start their family. Things didn't work out as they had planned, and she went back to substitute teaching. She was also very involved with her church and directed choirs, but she was often hurt by insensitive comments. Talking after school one day, we learned that we had much in common.

Sarah began the conversation with the query, "Don't you hate it when articles make us childless couples out to be selfish? I get very defensive about it. I want to call the authors up and say, 'Hey, I want kids. We just can't have them. Is that selfish?' "

"Yes," I replied. "Articles make it sound like just because we have material things and no children, we are selfish. Who doesn't have material things these days?"

Sarah continued, "I feel that I've gotten stuck with a lot of extra work because I'm a childless teacher. People figure I've got all sorts of time on my hands."

The topic of stereotypes came up again at one of our monthly bridge sessions. Karen said, "Doesn't it make you mad the way people think you'd never be a neat housekeeper if you had kids? I took care of three kids last fall, and was I ever proud when they noticed that my house still looked clean when they picked the kids up."

"Yes," Jan agreed. "My housekeeping skills haven't changed since we got our foster children."

I knew just what Karen and Jan were talking about. I was surprised, however, when Sharon told of thoughtless comments she had received: "A lot of people think I'm a career-oriented libber, which makes me less of a woman. They've also insinuated that we don't have children because my husband and I aren't very sure of our relationship."

"Is that ever awful!" said Sarah.

"I've had the same type of thing," stated Karen. "In fact, my neighbor asked a friend of mine if I was having an affair, simply because we don't have children."

"That's unbelievable!" responded Sarah. "Perhaps people are really jealous because we have other exciting things going. At least it seems that way to them."

Karen agreed. "I hear so many parents always complaining about their kids. They can hardly wait until the kids get back into school. I wonder why they had them in the first place. Sometimes—"

"But a lot of people just like to complain," interrupted Jan. "I complain about the weather constantly, but I really couldn't care less."

"True," replied Erica, "but remember Ann Landers' poll—70% of the parents responding said they wished they never had had children!"

A few weeks later Mary and I went to a lecture by Dr. William Glasser, noted psychiatrist and author of *Schools Without Failure*. He told of a session with a very depressed woman who was upset with him when he wouldn't allow her to tell about the cause of her depression. "Don't you want to find out why I'm depressed?" she yelled at him.

"Not really," he said. "I'm more interested in what you're going to do about it. What did you do today to solve the problem?"

How wise. Mary and I resolved to do something about our depression—to share more. But as I became less isolated, I found myself bitter and angry more often.

That summer on the tennis courts near my parents' cabin, I ran into a high school friend who greeted me with the old routine: "How are you? How many kids do you guys have now?" I fairly shouted back at her, "We don't have any kids." Craig later scolded me about my curt response, but I'd really had it with that question—the great assumption that everyone has children after X number of married years.

I also became increasingly angry at our church for being so family-oriented. Every Sunday the bulletin was filled with family activities, which infuriated me, even though I knew the majority of our church members had children. We quit being High League advisors, and I quit Churchwomen. I became involved in the Long-Range Planning Committee and some creative dramatics work with small groups.

I started to confide in my minister, who was now chairman of our adoption agency's board of directors. He was unaware of many of their adoption policies, and we frequently discussed them. He was always willing to listen and understand.

Christmas was again approaching, yet I felt none of my usual joy and enthusiasm. Everything seemed materialistic and child-oriented. Craig and I tried to concentrate on the true meaning of Christmas and to start our own nonchild-oriented Christmas customs. We invited other childless friends to be with us during the holidays and served everything *but* Scandinavian food: spaghetti one time, lobster another. We played tennis and went skiing rather than engaging in the typical Christmas activities. Christmas Eve we shared with Craig's mother and another couple and their parents. I couldn't stand being around a lot of children—nieces and nephews—and miraculously we were able to avoid it without offending anyone in the family.

I began to experience great physical pain, but refused to go to the doctor, certain that it was simply a reaction to the heavy dosage of medication and that it would pass. How I hated those Pills! But I would put up with anything if it would improve our chances of having a child.

I desperately wished my mother lived near us so I could talk with her. I had one close relative nearby, but whenever I mentioned my anger and frustrations or my pain, she implied that such problems were no more than what other people have. I should learn to keep my problems to myself, to have a "stiff upper lip." Again, isolation.

Sometimes, when I was very depressed, I'd try to think of two other people who had it worse than I. Earlier I'd tried to think of 10, but that was too hard because my own problems seemed immense. I felt God must be testing me: "Be glad for all God is planning for you. Be patient in trouble, and prayerful always," it says in Romans. So, ritualistically, I got up in the morning, read my Bible, and prayed for people on the prayer chain, even though many of their needs seemed much less critical than mine. My stubborn pride prevented me from putting my own name on the prayer chain. This was between Craig, God, and me.

No matter how hard I prayed, I didn't feel at peace with God, which added to my depression. I discussed this with my pastor and some of my guilt feelings were alleviated, but I still struggled with God's plan, desperately searching for peace.

My religious friends said, "It's God's will." That made it worse. God's will? Then maybe we shouldn't be pursuing the medical route. What was God's will? Here we were, seeking all possible means of having children. Were we taking things into our own hands? What had God planned for us? Should we just wait for God's great plan to unfold? Or did God give us talents to use to solve our own problems?

Everyone else thought we'd be great parents. Why

not God? I thought I was a good Christian. Did I have to work harder at it? Was I not reading my Bible regularly? Didn't Craig participate in church activities enough? Did we not give enough? I was brought up believing that we're saved through grace, not by works. Still, perhaps God wanted us to be of more service to him by not having children. Yet many "servants of God" had families. I searched in vain for answers.

I came to avoid religious discussions with my "newly born" Christian friends because they merely philosophized. They couldn't possibly know what I was going through. Craig gently chided me for expecting people to relate to my frame of reference, yet this is exactly what I did.

I was *angry* at almost everyone by now: at our adoption agency for their unfair policies, at my first doctor not discovering my endometriosis earlier, at God for giving children to parents who continually complain about them or can't care for them, at relatives and friends for not being empathetic and getting me to communicate, at Craig for not being upset about our childless state, and even at a local maternity shop for making "pregnant pretty" a household phrase in our city.

In spite of, or perhaps because of, my fluctuations between depression and anger, Craig and I began to communicate more, to really talk together. Maybe this was one of God's hidden plans for us, as I had always wished Craig would open up more on personal matters. Although I came from a home where we communicated freely and openly, Craig's background was somewhat different. Now, however, we spent many evenings just talking, becoming closer than ever before.

We decided to forego the traditional family gathering at Easter and to take a trip to Galena, Illinois, the antique capitol of the Midwest. That weekend, however, we had a blizzard. "Just my luck," I complained bitterly. "Nothing seems to go right anymore." Undaunted, Craig suggested we spend the weekend at a nearby posh hotel. The luxurious, extravagant weekend was excellent therapy, as Craig must have known it would be. I felt better, but still not like the Kaye of old.

I dreaded returning to school after vacation. Teaching was getting me down. By now I had taught almost eight years, and I felt drained. I had a sixth grade class, and discipline problems were getting worse. The kids had little respect for authority and seemed unappreciative of the special things I planned for them. I resented teaching other people's children and hated it when friends asked, "Are you *still* teaching?" I had always enjoyed teaching and felt I was a creative, effective teacher, but now I was negative about my profession. My anger came out at the children, my colleagues, the district, and the entire school system. Was this related to my medication, my infertility, or "the times?" I wasn't sure. I just knew I had to get out.

Then I'd consider the security of the job and the extra income. We had moved to our second home, with increased payments and expenses, so giving up the second salary would be difficult. And what would I do with myself? I knew how sorry Sarah was that she had quit teaching—now she could only get substitute work.

Still, was it fair to stay in teaching feeling the way I did? I just couldn't decide.

Later that spring Craig and I took our trip to Galena, a quaint historic town. We agreed to forget our problems and simply enjoy each other, and for a while the beautiful rolling hills and valleys did make me forget. But not for long. I was obsessed with our infertility.

One night after an elegant dinner, I cried hysterically because I felt so worthless. I wasn't a mother; I was a failure. I wasn't a good teacher anymore; I was a failure. I wasn't a good wife, as I couldn't give Craig a child and I couldn't even let him enjoy his vacation; I was a failure. I wasn't a good daughter, as I couldn't give my parents a grandchild; I was a failure. A total failure as a woman and a human. What purpose did I have, anyway?

To make matters worse, Mother's Day was approaching. I resented the church for glorifying motherhood. I hated the TV ads depicting mothers and daughters with long, flowing, golden hair running through fields and mothers powdering their babies' round little bottoms. Even shampooing hair was visualized as a partnership between mother and daughter. I was so depressed I couldn't force myself to buy a present for my mother or mother-in-law, or even send them cards. Instead I wrote a lengthy letter to Ann Landers, expressing my resentment toward Mother's Day.

What did I have to look forward to? Would I get pregnant after I went off the Pill? Would adoption ever come through? We began to consider applying at the agency Bob and Diane were going through, but we learned there was little hope of receiving a Caucasian infant and, further, it is "against the rules" to have your name in with more than one agency. We feared we might be dropped by our first agency if we applied with a second. "As if the social worker would ever bother to check it out," I thought bitterly. "They don't even know we exist half the time."

Some friends suggested we try private adoption, but, unfortunately, in our state private adoption was illegal. True, many people were doing it, but it was terribly expensive, besides being against the law. There was also the possibility of the grey market and the black market, but we wanted no part of anything illegal. Although by now we were firmly convinced we had placed our names with the wrong agency, we stayed with it, Craig patiently, I impatiently.

One way to reduce the waiting time to receive a child would be to adopt a child of another race. Of course, we would have to remove our name from the waiting list for a Caucasian child—you couldn't be on two lists at the same time. Craig and I discussed the topic more and more frequently. Although I was open to a child of any race, Craig argued that we didn't have many non-Caucasian friends, and that it would be hard enough to adjust to becoming parents without the added problems of adopting a child from a minority group.

I finally agreed to wait for a Caucasian child, but I felt guilty and selfish about the decision. Many groups were oriented to adoption of racially mixed children, and by now many of our friends, some with adopted racially mixed children themselves, knew we were trying to adopt. Somehow I felt we had to justify our decision to wait for a Caucasian child. But why should we not want a child as much like us as possible? Isn't that typical? Don't we all get indoctrinated early in life that we will have children like ourselves someday? Still, I was haunted by the possibility that our decision might mean we would end up with *no* child. What then? It all seemed so hopeless.

One afternoon shortly after we made this decision, the phone rang and Diane, breathless, exclaimed, "Kaye, we have our boy! His name is Matthew. He's here, Kaye! You've got to come over right away." Emotions came flooding. A shiver of excitement and joy raced through me. I was as happy for them as they would have been for us—momentarily. Then followed one of the hardest days I've ever lived through. I went right over to their house and hugged them and their new son. I role-played myself through the endless afternoon, holding their cooing baby and assisting in picture-taking sessions.

Diane must have known it was hard on me. We had discussed what this day would be like for the other. She kept asking, "Are you sure you're all right?"

"Yes," I assured her, but my heart ached with emptiness. My closest friend who could identify with infertility had just become a mother and was off into the world of parenthood. Could she ever again really feel the hurt of infertility?

The next week I met a friend who told me about a couple who had also just received a child through our adoption agency. "I'm so thrilled for them. They had such a difficult time, waiting two whole years." I couldn't believe what I had heard. They had their name in for only two years? Our name had been in for five! I called up our social worker and furiously asked if this was true. The only response I received was that each individual case was handled differently, and that the information was confidential. I wanted to scream at that social worker, but I was afraid she'd think I was foolish, unstable, or even neurotic. "Patience, Kaye, patience," I told myself. "Thank you," I murmured, and glumly hung up.

Shortly after that my vocal neighbor got her third child from our adoption agency. She called me to come over about a week after the little girl arrived. Near exhaustion and ill, she said flatly, "The baby is such a handful, I think I should return her to the agency."

Return the child? I couldn't believe it. Anger and bitterness again overwhelmed me. Where was God's justice? Where? Why couldn't this little girl have been ours?

When the anger subsided, I was more depressed than ever. Without a child, I felt I couldn't be the "total woman" I thought I should be. My feelings of inadequacy were magnified every time I saw a pregnant friend.

The crowning blow came when my youngest sister became pregnant. I hit an all-time low. I would not be the one to give my parents their first grandchild. Although they had never asked us to do this, we had wanted to. And now I was jealous of my sister. We had become very close since her marriage, but I couldn't bear this. I didn't want to ruin her happiness by letting her know my feelings. I had to become closed, cool, and uncommunicative, or fall apart.

I imagined my parents and their friends all knew Craig and I couldn't "make the grade" and pitied us. I envisioned them saying, "Poor Kaye, this must really be hard on her." But no one ever confronted me with what was most obviously on my mind, not even my parents, which was difficult to understand and accept. If they weren't aware of my feelings, it was because I acted so indifferently about the whole thing, hiding my true self from those who should know me best.

Night after night, I cried myself to sleep. Craig would tell me over and over that I was not a failure. I asked what had I done to show that I was not a failure? What had I accomplished? He gave many answers, but none registered. They were all meaningless. I was a failure because I hadn't accomplished what *I* wanted to do, and no one understood, not even God.

It was then that I thought of suicide—really contemplated it. I didn't admit that to anyone. I knew it would flash neon signs of total instability to my friends, family—and adoption agency. I told Craig I couldn't go on any more, but I don't think he believed I would go so far as to commit suicide, although he was seriously concerned about my depression.

People can talk glibly about what a sin it is to commit suicide, but I did not believe that. I felt it would be best for everyone concerned, an act of love and compassion. It seemed the most unselfish thing I could do—

sparing others from having to be with such a pitiable person as I.

One night I felt I simply could not face another day. Pills, poisons, and car accidents kept flashing through my mind, and then the peace of death and the joy of heaven. Through all these visions, however, I kept hearing Craig's words: "I love you, Kaye. You cannot fail at that over which you have no control."

I loved Craig deeply and knew he was right. I had no real control over whether I could get pregnant or whether the adoption agency would ever place a child with us. I turned to my Bible and hoped to find strength to continue. God's words provided the direction I sought:

For to me, living means opportunities for Christ, and dying— well, that's better yet! But if living will give me more opportunities to win people to Christ, then I really don't know which is better, to live or die! Sometimes I want to live and other times I don't, for I long to go with Christ. How much happier for *me* than being here. But the fact is that I can be of more help to *you* by staying. (Phil. 1:21-24 LB).

I drew a bold line under the last sentence in the passage and resolved to shake my depression. It had been more than nine months since I'd begun taking the Pill again. I was up to five a day and was an emotional and physical wreck. I made an appointment to see the doctor and asked to be taken off the Pill. He willingly agreed. Now the wait.

I became deeply involved in creative dramatics and tried to keep my mind off whether or not I would become pregnant. Although time seemed to drag on interminably, it was passing faster than I realized. Suddenly I was facing my 30th birthday. I dreaded the day, and was thankful when Diane and Bob invited Craig and me out to dinner and then to the theatre to watch a mime perform. Good friends, good food, and good entertainment helped to soften the blow.

Although I grew up believing I would have my family completed by the time I was 30, my 30th birthday had come and gone, and still we had no children. Now I began to hear my friends talk about starting their family before they were 35. But I did not plan to be like Sarah who conceived her first child when she was 90!

We often make too much of age, yet it is a reality, and it was especially real to us because of our adoption agency's age policy. I thought the policy was unreasonable. Although most couples have their full families by 30, everyone is different. I read once that older couples make *better* parents, because they have had so many experiences and are ready to settle down to serious parenting. Yet, maybe the image of serious parenting is all wrong, too. Who can say at what age good parents are made and from what experiences they come?

As I pondered the question of age, I decided it was largely a state of mind. I knew 30-year-olds who acted and talked as if they were 80, and vice versa. A poem someone sent to me entitled "Youth" echoed my thoughts. I added it to the collection on my refrigerator door to help keep my spirits up. Two lines were especially encouraging:

Youth is not a time of life, it is a state of mind, . . .
You are as young as your faith and as old as your doubts.

Now that I was off the Pill, there was renewed hope that I might become pregnant any day. We waited, and waited, and waited, and waited, but nothing happened. Nine months of misery for nothing!

Only one hope remained—artificial insemination. This can be done with the husband's sperm or with that of a donor. We were fortunate; we could use Craig's sperm, and artificial insemination was done in our city. Some people have to wait a year to get a donor, and then have to drive to another town or state and stay for a week at phenomenal expense.

Still, the decision to undergo artificial insemination was difficult, even with Craig as the donor. If God wanted me to become pregnant, would we have to go this far? Was this taking things into our own hands? Or does God help those who help themselves?

I once heard a woman who had conceived her family naturally criticize a physician who was transplanting the eggs from one female to another by saying: "Aren't you playing God, taking life into your own hands?" The doctor simply replied, "And what will you do if your child has leukemia? Leave it to the will of God? Or will you pursue the best medical services available?" We decided to try artificial insemination.

Our sessions were always scheduled when it was least convenient. I would collect the sperm at home and drive to the clinic with a cupful carefully tucked in my bra to keep it as near to body temperature as possible. The traffic would be at its worst; it would be snowing; Craig would be scheduled for a meeting; I'd have company coming in. Something, always something. We never told anyone what we were doing; it was just too personal.

Artificial insemination was cold, unloving, sterile, and extremely difficult emotionally. My religious beliefs made it even worse, because I feared trying to take over God's will. We went through three sessions, and after each I would eagerly look forward to the next month and no Big Red. But Big Red always came, and with it deep depression.

Finally we agreed we could no longer go on with this. We had done more than most. This was it, at least for now. At my next appointment I told the doctor we wanted to discontinue artificial insemination, and then I totally broke down, crying uncontrollably. Five straight mornings of artificial insemination had left me ready to break. The doctor put his hand on my shoulder and asked sternly, "Can't you *cope* anymore?"

"Cope! Cope!" I screamed back. "That's all I've been doing for five years. I'm sick of trying to cope!"

"Do you think you need to see a psychiatrist?"

His reply left me silent. Since my sister Mary had been institutionalized off and on throughout most of her adult life, the fear of going crazy was very real to me. Logic quickly returned. "Kaye, you've gone too far this time. He thinks you're crazy. You'd better shape up, and fast."

I rejected the offer to see a psychiatrist. I knew I must learn to cope with our reality—our infertility. I must put my trust in God and accept my life.

6

Coping

Strength comes from struggle; weakness from ease
—B. C. Forbes

As I left the doctor's office that bright, crisp winter morning, tears were streaming down my cheeks. In despair, I intended to tell Craig if this session didn't prove to be fruitful, literally, I would give up on all future sessions, no matter what my doctor advised.

I was walking back to the parking lot, softly sobbing, "Cope, cope," when suddenly the sun's rays were captured in the stained-glass windows of a church nearby. The windows shone with such intensity that I stood spellbound. The light was of such brilliance that the church seemed to overflow with the love and warmth of the Holy Spirit.

It had actually happened—a sign from God showing me that a light *was* guiding my way through life, a sign that surely he would give me strength in my time of need. But I, too, must give strength to others when I could. The light was a commandment from God to do something important with my life.

As I drove home wondering what I could do for others, I was suddenly inspired, indeed, compelled, to write a book about infertility, a book offering others comfort in their crisis. I had complained bitterly about the lack of books on the subject. I had searched the libraries and agencies for reading material, but everything I found was written by a Ph.D. in medicine, undecipherable to me. I could do something about it.

When I got home, I laid out the outline for the chapters I'd include. Everything came together so easily, I was amazed. I was certain God was leading me. However, having never experienced anything like this before, I didn't mention it to anyone for fear I would be accused of being overly dramatic.

I stopped judging God's ways. I'd been driving myself crazy with questions about why others became pregnant or were able to adopt while we couldn't. Now, through a leap of faith, I realized things would work out for the best. "Let God's will be done," I thought to myself.

That evening I told Craig of my plan to write a book. He paused a minute, probably thinking, "I wonder what she'll be feeling like next week. But at least she seems more enthusiastic than she has been for months." He answered, "Great, I think you should."

The next day I received a letter from my mom, with a poem enclosed she thought I'd like:

Accept your womanhood, my daughter, and rejoice in it.
It is your glory that you are a woman, for that is why
    he loves you, he whom you love.
Be gentle, be wise, as a woman is gentle and wise.
Be ardent and love with a woman's ardor.
Through your love, teach him what it means to be a man,
    a noble man, a strong man.
Believe in him, for only through your belief can he
    believe in himself.
In your secret heart, man and woman, we long above all
    else to know that the other, the one we love,
    knows what we are and believes in what we can be.
Is this not romance?
Yes, and the highest romance, investing the smallest
    detail of life with the color of joy.

Another godsend. I taped it to the refrigerator and vowed that I would accept my womanhood. "OK, look out world, I'm ready to cope. I'm going to get through this infertility crisis once and for all."

I began to believe in Craig's philosophy that you cannot fail at that over which you have no control. All right. We had taken control of what we could. We had sought out the best medical care, and we had sought adoption. What else could we do but wait, pray, and trust the Lord?

The decision to stop artificial insemination lifted a great burden from me. If I did get pregnant, wonderful. If not, we would eventually have our adopted child. So on with it.

I decided from this point on that when I didn't like something I'd do something about it rather than simply complain. The first thing I had to do was look squarely at what I wanted to do with my life. Teaching was no longer satisfying. What I felt to be permissive, open education and lack of respect from students and parents was getting harder to take every year. A teacher influences so many lives, and feeling as I did, I could do more harm than good. I was "burned out" on teaching. "Take that leave of absence you've earned after seven years," I said to myself. And that's exactly what I did.

I had no idea what I'd do that fall, but I became more engrossed in homemaking and took up many sewing and craft projects. Lanna and Rick were back from Europe, looking for a place to set up Rick's dental practice. They were considering Flagstaff, Arizona, and planned to drive down there to check it out. They had three children by then, and they asked us if we'd consider taking care of two of them while they were gone.

I readily agreed, eager to get to know their two boys, ages 9 months and 21 months. This would give me some experience at mothering and allow me to view family life more realistically. Maybe I wasn't cut out for it. Craig thought it would be fun too. Some of our friends, however, weren't optimistic. "Both of them?" "Are you kidding?" "Boy, are you in for it."

The boys came, and although they were a handful, I enjoyed every minute, except for an occasional diaperful. When Lanna and Rick returned two weeks later, Todd was playing outside with some neighbors and Dane was pulling things out of my dresser drawers. Trailings of kids' muss led throughout the house.

I greeted Lanna and Rick with tears. I had grown to

love the boys in those two short weeks and dreaded the thought of seeing them go. Lanna guessed what I was going through, and we cried our farewells.

Not long after that, Craig and I enrolled in a foster care program with our county government. At the challenging six-week training session, we learned that foster care is a satisfying alternative for many childless couples and for many couples with children. Foster parents can help children cope with not having parents or having parents who can't or won't take care of them. They can provide a home for a child whose mother is hospitalized for alcoholism, a child whose parents are abusive, a child who has been taken care of by aging grandparents who can no longer manage the responsibility. For such children, foster parents can provide the love and understanding so critical to normal growth and development.

I had two friends who were continuously involved in foster care, and their experiences were very rewarding. One told me, "I've always wanted to have a lot of kids around, since I came from a small family and felt I really missed out. We became concerned with the social pressure to limit our family, so for us foster children were the solution. There's nothing I'd rather do than play with my kids—a lot of them. Sometimes it's hectic. Once Vicki, our foster daughter, invited 17 relatives to our home on her birthday—unbeknownst to me. But I loved it."

Another foster parent, herself a former foster child, said, "Now that I'm a parent myself, I realize more than ever the influence my foster parents had on my life. I carried their love and encouragement with me even when I went back home. I can't help but think my own son will be happier because of their influence."

I was eager to find out what our first experience as foster parents would be, what kind of child would join our home. But I was also preparing for a new career: interior design. I was deeply engrossed in my studies when, unexpectedly, we received a phone call from Foster Care. Would we be willing to take a three-year-old boy with severe problems?

When it came right down to it, I wasn't sure. I described the situation to my friend who worked with foster children and who'd had a three-year-old. She told me that I'd be up against a lot for our first experience and to consider the pros and cons carefully.

I was in a quandary. I knew clearly that my heart wasn't in it, yet I thought this was something I should be doing. After much thought I realized I'd gone into this program for the wrong reasons. I wanted to be a foster parent to see if I could cope with parenting once I was older than 30. I also hoped to be lucky enough to get a foster child we would be able to adopt. My reasons were selfish, not child-oriented. We had to say no.

Although I was not over my depression with infertility, I began coping fairly well. My enthusiasm for life was returning. I worked diligently on my book— excellent therapy. As I put my thoughts in writing, I was able to look at infertility more objectively, at least in spurts.

I learned from Dr. Elisabeth Kubler-Ross's *On Death and Dying* (Macmillan, 1969) that one goes through certain stages when experiencing a life crisis. I had definitely experienced the first stage: *isolation*. I'd felt I was the only one in the world who was infertile. I had also been through the second stage: *anger and resentment*. I was angry at everyone for not understanding that I was suffering, and I resented everyone who had children. And I had been through the third stage: *depression*. I might have attempted suicide if it had not been for my love of Craig. It seemed I was now in the fourth and final stage: *coping and resolution*. I was learning to accept life for what it was, whatever it had to offer. Writing my book was helping me cope and helping me to see myself more clearly.

I had experienced firsthand the truth embodied in Gloria Evans's parable *The Wall* (Word Books, 1977) which shows how people protect themselves by building walls to help them deal comfortably with others. Each stone in the wall fills a need, yet the stones often block honest communication. Sometimes our walls become so high no one can get inside. Often in our isolation we begin to see our imperfections, our various stones of pride, jealousy, anger, impatience, and guilt.

Such withdrawal is generally an attempt to be safe. Infertile people often endure painful comments, but it is sometimes our own fault because we do not know how to take down our safe walls. None of us probably intended to build our walls so high, but once they're built, it is a challenge for others to reach us. We have to let our hurt be known, to tell people what hurts and what helps. This involves risk, because the result may be the last thing we want or need—pity. That is only more hurt. What we want is empathy, for others to understand our wall and our need for it.

The parable concludes with a penetration of the wall by a greater spirit, the spirit of love, compassion, and power which helps us take down our walls and open our hearts. We all need understanding and love, and they can only occur through honest communication. However, we must also understand the walls of others. Not everyone knows how to communicate our way. It is here we must pray for strength from God so we do not let other people's walls cause us to build our own walls higher. We must learn to deal with rejection of our ideas without feeling personally rejected.

I began looking at childless and childfree living more rationally and discussing it with friends who were in the same quandary as Craig and I. Following one of our monthly bridge get-togethers, Sandy said, "We're still undecided about having children. I never even thought about it until I was 30. Now we can't put the decision off any longer. But I'm happy, and I like my career. I'd like to pursue administration, and can't see being a parent too. Still, we're not selfish, and I think we'd be good parents. I don't want to face 35 and then start thinking, 'Hey, we should start our family.' But I think about it only when we've been with close friends who have kids. I'm curious to know if I can even have children. Isn't that a horrid reason for having them?"

"I don't think that's unusual," responded Carolyn. "I'm sure many of us wonder about our fertility. And I'm concerned with the age factor, too. My mother had me when she was 38 and went through her menopause when I was a teenager. We both almost had nervous breakdowns. I'd never start having kids at that late stage."

"That reminds me of what happened at work one day," said Carolyn. "Everyone was exclaiming because Martha Nelson was having a baby. 'Isn't it wonderful?' they all said. 'What's so wonderful about that?' I asked. A hush fell over the room, and finally Jean Sorenson said in a soft, hushed voice, 'If you were 50 and had been trying for 25 years, you'd think it was wonderful, too.' I just about sank through the floor. Even after that experience, I still refuse to congratulate anyone who says they're expecting because I feel the environmental impact so strongly. We'll be starving worldwide in the not-too-distant future. I wonder if I want a child of mine growing up in this world."

"Yes," concurred Erica. "I went to a meeting of NON, a very impressive group of people with a definite commitment to not having children. Many of them had been sterilized. It was interesting, yet frightening. Here were all these vital people, very educated, able to afford children, and they aren't having any. It seems more and more only the uneducated and the poor are having babies, and getting money from the government to take care of them. In a democracy, this scares me."

"Wait a minute," Sharon interrupted. "When we start running down people with kids, we're just as bad in our stereotyping of them."

"But some people make children their whole life," said Sara. "I know women who are only people through their kids. And financially it's a big responsibility to have children."

"That's for sure," agreed Erica. "We have a lot of expenses now. We're planning so we'll be financially prepared and there won't be a lot of pressure. We'll have our family in a year or so."

That was exactly what Craig and I had thought. "What if you can't get pregnant?" I asked gently.

"That doesn't bother me," responded Erica. "As much as I want children, if I learned tomorrow I couldn't, I'd just say, 'That's the way it is.' We have a very happy marriage and a child might interfere with that."

"Ignorance *is* bliss," I thought to myself. "You don't really know how you'll feel until it actually happens to you.

"Still," I said aloud, "although choosing to be child-*free* is one way to resolve infertility, to be truly child-free, you must have the choice: otherwise it may become an excuse for being child*less*."

That winter I went to stay with Ruth and their new baby Kirsten for a week. Ruth's fantastic empathy allowed us to become close again. She knew just how to get me to open up, and we had many long talks, sharing feelings on infertility and coping with various crises that life brings. I was so grateful I had her. I felt no bitterness toward her and Kirsten, yet if we hadn't talked so openly, wounds could have festered.

"Why did you have a child so easily?" I asked. I learned that her delivery had been very painful and that having a child always involves some struggle, either physical or emotional. "Why did everything work out so perfectly in your marriage?" I asked, only to learn that they had their problems, like all married couples. I shared with Ruth my feelings about Mom and Dad not seeming to care about my emptiness at being childless. Ruth said they cared deeply, but were afraid to approach the subject because I had become so defensive. They were aware that too much questioning by parents can cut off the channels of communication. They were trying to be unmeddling in-laws rather than "outlaws."

When Ruth asked if we'd be godparents for Kirsten, I eagerly accepted. We made plans for a trip to Atlanta a week before Palm Sunday, the day scheduled for the baptism. This would give Craig and me a chance to tell my parents about our plans for a family, to spend time with them alone. We also planned to spend a few days vacationing on our own. Ruth and Jack would arrive two days before Palm Sunday.

I was looking forward to the trip, eager to tell my parents about my new studies and work in interior design. Still, I was apprehensive. I imagined the excitement the visit of my parents' first grandchild would cause, and I wasn't sure how well I would handle it.

I desperately wanted to regain the closeness with my parents that comes through total, open communication. I remembered my mother telling me after we were married that it was so much fun now that we were on the same level and could discuss adult topics; it was like having a new friend. I really wanted to feel that way with her, yet I knew I would be battling with pride. Having my book to talk about would help. I couldn't wait to tell her about the information I'd uncovered in my research.

Since my first search for appropriate reading material, I had found some new books, but still none that addressed the childless couple and how to cope with infertility. I had come to understand what infertility is and, equally important, what it is not. Reputable dictionaries provided little help. For example, *Webster's New World Dictionary* defines *infertile* as "not fertile, not productive, barren." The synonym given is *sterile.* This may be acceptable for referring to a desert, but not for referring to people.

In contrast, *Saunders Medical Dictionary* (24th edition) defines *infertility* as "absence of the ability to conceive or to induce conception." Most physicians carry this definition one step further and define infertility as "the inability to conceive a pregnancy after a year or more of regular sexual relations without contraception, or the inability to carry pregnancies to a live birth." The term *sterility* is reserved for permanent, incurable infertility. A woman who has had a hysterectomy is sterile.

Fortunately, infertility is not an absolute. Many myths about infertility need to be dispelled. Menning notes several such myths*:

1. *Infertility is not a "female condition."* In almost half of all cases, the man is involved in the infertility problem. A breakdown of the causes of infertility reveals that women

---

* Barbara Eck Menning, *Infertility: A Guide for the Childless Couple,* © 1977, p. 5. Reprinted by permission of Prentice-Hall, Inc., Englewood Cliffs, New Jersey.

have the problem in 40 percent of the cases, men have the problem in 40 percent of the cases, and the couple share a problem in the remaining 20 percent of the cases.

2. *Infertility is not usually due to psychological factors.* A *physical* problem is found in 90 percent of all cases that have been thoroughly investigated by a qualified doctor. The remaining 10 percent may have a problem that cannot be diagnosed with current technology.

3. *Infertility is not incurable.* Over 50 percent of those couples who enter a proper investigation of their problem will respond to treatment and conceive. Compare this to the "spontaneous cure rate" (pregnancy without a doctor's help) of only 5 percent in those couples who have been infertile over one year.

4. *Infertility is not a sexual disorder.* In the vast majority of cases, infertility has nothing to do with ability to perform sexual relations. Infertile men and women are capable of experiencing the same spectrum of physical and emotional responses in sexual relations that other couples do.

5. *It is not immoral or irresponsible to want to bear children and to work at it.* Zero Population Growth is an admirable cause, but a couple should not feel guilty because they want a child and are working on it. ZPG means that each couple has the right to two children to replace themselves. Those who wish to remain childfree or raise single children have the right to do so. Infertility, for those who desire children, represents a denial of the right to choose.

I also discovered that infertility is becoming more common. More than 10 million people in the United States alone are experiencing infertility. I learned that causes of infertility are varied and complex. Often the reason is medical. For example, the increase in venereal disease is one cause. In addition, some forms of birth control are now thought to increase the possibility of infertility. The trend toward delaying marriage and childbearing is another reason for the increase in infertility.

I also discovered opposing views on motherhood as a woman's primary function in life. I had always felt motherhood *was* woman's primary function; that's why I suffered so. That's also why the media bothered me so greatly; it showed me as being out of the mainstream. Elizabeth Whelan's *A Baby . . . Maybe* (Bobbs-Merrill, 1975) cited a variety of experts on "motherhood," some concurring with what I'd always believed:

Erik Erikson, in his essay "Woman and the Inner Space," clearly concurs with Freud on the idea that reproduction is the woman's primary role in life. The woman who does not satisfy her innate need to fill her inner space, or uterus, with embryotic tissue is likely to be frustrated or neurotic. . . . "Women especially, but not exclusively, are apt to feel that they are frustrated in something essential if they do not produce children. . . ." You get funny. . . . You might even get sick. You stagnate.

But then, Whalen cites other experts who disagree with this view of motherhood:

"Motherhood . . . a biological destiny? Forget biology!" says sociologist/author Dr. Jessie Bernard. "If it were biology, people would die from not doing it."

"Women don't need to be mothers, any more than they need spaghetti," claims Dr. Richard Rabkin, a New York psychiatrist. "But if you're in a world where everyone is eating spaghetti thinking they need it and want it, you will think so too."

I found these views comforting. Maybe motherhood is not our primary function. What about spouses, friends, and work? I had found other goals for my life. I knew I had something to offer, and it didn't have to be motherhood and family. Yet self-acceptance comes only after a long, slow process.

David and Ruth Kirk ("The Challenge of Change") concur that women have a great deal of difficulty accepting infertility. They note that infertile women have to depend on assistance from outsiders such as doctors and agencies, which are often too busy counseling the unwed mother to have time for the *wedded unmother*.

A second difficulty Kirk and Kirk note is the lack of a dependable timetable. Our adoption agency had been telling us for the last four years that our name would come to the top of the waiting list in two years, but so far it had not.

A third difficulty is accepting that you won't have a child born to you. Professional "help" in accepting this fact often consists of comments such as, "We have to make the best of things" and "You'll love an adopted child just as much as if it were your own." Such cliches are not very helpful for those suffering the heartbreak of infertility. I was encouraged by Kirk and Kirk's views and I renewed in my efforts to write this book as one means of helping others accept infertility. I was also eager to share all my new findings with my parents.

My expectations of the trip to Atlanta were high. I was definitely learning to cope with my life crisis through a new profession, a new project to help others, and renewed faith in God. I finally knew who I was and what I believed in, and I was at peace. I believed God cared for me, that I was precious to him, and that he would take care of my needs. I was looking forward to whatever life might hold.

7

Resolution

We must take life as we find it
and improve it as we can.

—Lloyd Garrison

In making final preparations for our trip to Atlanta, I checked the refrigerator to be sure nothing was there that would spoil. I lingered to read some of the quotations taped on the door:

The person who prides himself on having the courage to say what he thinks should be sure he thinks.—Anonymous

A philosopher is a person who knows just what to do until it happens to him.—Henry Hasse

I wish all my problems had happened when I was 17 and knew all the answers.—Kaye

What a pity human beings can't exchange problems. Everyone knows exactly how to solve the other fellow's.—Olin Miller

Things could be worse. Suppose they published your errors daily like they do for baseball players.—Anonymous

If you are all wrapped up in yourself, you are overdressed.—Anonymous

Accept your womanhood. . . .

This mixture of lightness and seriousness matched my mood exactly. I was ready for a fun vacation, for enjoying Craig's companionship and new surroundings, for sharing with my family. This vacation would not be marred with tears and self-pity.

Craig and I boarded the plane for Atlanta, laughing and joking together. When we arrived, my mother was eager to show us the spots of local color they had discovered. One particular favorite was a lake cabin of friends who kindly loaned it to us for the weekend. We immediately fell in love with the secluded, woodsy hideaway. After eating and getting into comfy clothes, I looked forward to our usual talks lasting into the late hours, but for some reason no one said much. Dad was exhausted from long hours of counseling, and I was becoming tense about what we would discuss and about the visit of their first grandchild. Craig was relaxed, but didn't initiate any earthshaking discussion. It was a completely uneventful evening, filled with small talk. Much to my disappointment, we all retired early.

Craig and I left the next morning for a week's vacation at Myrtle Beach. I had lost the exuberance I'd felt when we boarded the plane in Minneapolis. Craig, raring to go for a fun-filled week, disliked the early tell-tale signs he was getting from me. I knew I should lick my foul mood, but somehow I couldn't. All week I dreaded the upcoming baptism, believing that friends and family alike would be perceiving me as the over-30 daughter who was infertile and childless.

I was experiencing the fact that the stages of a life crisis do not progress in textbook sequence. I had regressed to deep depression and knew I must once again cope. Our vacation was "nice." The scenery was breathtaking, the tennis fun, and the food fantastic, but I couldn't really enjoy any of it. Craig, as always, was cheerful, energetic, and continuously on the go, taking me sightseeing and shopping. We bought a large hurricane lamp in one little town, and the decorator side of me was thrilled. I couldn't wait to take it home and put it in a place of honor on our dining room table.

We returned to Atlanta the same day Ruth, Jack, and Kirsten were due. Their plane was late and my parents, usually so calm, were in a tizzy over the delay. I resented their anxiety. I imagined it all stemmed from excitement over their new grandchild's arrival. "They'd never make such a fuss if it was just Craig and I arriving," I thought bitterly.

After what seemed an eternity, they arrived to be greeted with a round of hugs, kisses, and a chorus of "Isn't she precious?" as we oohed and aahed over Kirsten. But my heart ached that it wasn't Craig and me giving such joy to my mom and dad. My worst fears were being realized. I knew I couldn't hold back the tears, so I prayed they would be interpreted as tears of happiness.

We all piled into the car and went to my folks' home to make final preparations for the next day's baptism. I went to bed heartsick, hoping my feelings of hurt, frustration, and worthlessness would pass by morning. But when I awoke, they were still there. How could I take part in the ceremony feeling so depressed? I dreaded the appearance in front of the church congregation. Whenever I sat in church with my mother while my father was preaching, I felt deeply emotional. Today would be especially difficult.

I told Craig I didn't think I could take it. The only thing stopping me from telling Ruth and Jack that I couldn't be Kirsten's godmother was that I knew it would ruin their day and my parents' day too. I just couldn't be that selfish. Still, I didn't think I could stand up in church and not break down publicly, and I couldn't handle that either. Craig, knowing I was serious, tried everything to keep me from backing out. Humor finally did it. "Kaye," he told me, "if you don't shape up, I'll break our hurricane lamp in a million pieces." That sounded so funny coming from Craig, always so easygoing, that I couldn't help but smile. Any time that morning I looked as if I might break down, Craig whispered into my ear, "Where's that lamp?"

Although a few tears escaped at the service, it was nothing like I had imagined. I was relieved when the baptism was over, but I desperately wished my mother or father had come up to me sometime during the day, put their arms around me, and said something, anything, to let me know they understood what I was going through. When our plane left for Minneapolis that evening, I was filled with anger and resentment toward my parents for not getting me to open up, for not realizing that I was too stubborn and proud to bring up what was on my mind.

My mother wrote to us shortly after our return:

Dear Kaye and Craig,

So many thoughts come crowding in. We are enjoying having Kirsten here for the first time, and yet there is not complete joy. Our hearts ache knowing that as yet your hopes are not completely fulfilled. I guess life will never have a completeness while we are strangers and pilgrims "here below." Something in us always longs for "our" children, so we refrain from showing our real feelings for fear we make them feel bound instead of free from us. None of this makes real sense, only we loved your visit. Thanks for coming. We love you both very much.

Love,
Mom and Dad

My vision clouded, a lump rose in my throat, and the tears began to flow. Why hadn't things been discussed when we were there? They obviously *did* know my thoughts. Why didn't we talk? As the hurt subsided, resentment again welled up. Why didn't they have the strength to discuss this with me face to face? They seemed phony, wrapped up in games people play. But hadn't I done the same thing? I resolved to get my feelings into the open, to write it all down and send it to them, no matter what the consequences:

Dear Mom and Dad,

You can't imagine the flood of emotions I went through upon reading your letter. Why is it that people who love each other so much don't communicate their feelings openly and honestly when they're together but have to do it through letters? You said once early in the week of our stay how great it is to know your children are raised and don't need their parents anymore. You're wrong. Children always need their parents in some way.

I needed you both so much last week and so many other times this past year. I wanted so badly to have a good, open, heart-to-heart talk, the four of us. I hoped Lake Nexter would do it, a serene time alone, away from the city, the phone, and drop-in company. I'm not blaming you for not trying to open us up; it's equally our fault, my fault. I just became extremely stubborn. Although I don't normally consider myself stubborn, I've learned that people don't like to have others talk about their problems, so I didn't.

I once felt so very close to you both; I could always go to you to talk whenever I needed. What's happened to us? I hear you tell about staying up with others and their problems until the wee hours in the morning, but when we were together, we were in bed by nine o'clock. That really hurt. Again, I'm not blaming either of you. It's so often true in one's vocation; we are in the social ministries and very professional in helping others, but it's so difficult to reach our very own loved ones.

Mom, I needed you so much the night you stayed over with me alone before going to see Ruth's new baby. I needed some words like "I know how this must be affecting you." I wanted so badly to go into your room and let everything out, but my stubborn pride prevented me. I cried myself to sleep, softly for fear you'd hear my grief. I felt that since you were the mother, older and wiser, you should understand me better than I could understand myself. I probably needed you even more than Ruth did that week.

I needed you, too, Dad, this past week. I love our "heavy"

discussions, and I love hearing your sermons. Do you know what emotions I experience every time I hear you preach? I had all I could do to get through each Sunday's service, especially Kirsten's baptism. Your sermon was outstanding, Dad, and said so many things to me personally. Some time I'll share these feelings if you ask me. You see, I feel I've never really lived up to your expectations; I feel like such a failure in your eyes. Please don't blame yourself for doing anything to cause this; you haven't. I'm just sometimes super-sensitive. It's my own fault. But why do we have to be so outwardly busy? Why can't we take time to sense the needs and feelings of those closest to us?

Mother, your letter is a real keeper. It will go into my secret compartment to read when I need a lift. "Life will never have a completeness while we are strangers and pilgrims 'here below.'" I guess that's my biggest difficulty now. I've prayed so long for opportunities to give my life completeness. I know I analyze everything too deeply—at least that's what Craig says—but that's my nature, and there isn't a whole lot I can do about it. "Accept your womanhood, my daughter, and rejoice in it." Perhaps that is what I'm searching for, a way to do it now.

You said in your letter how much you were looking forward to having Kirsten there for the first time, and yet "there is never complete joy because our hearts ache knowing that as yet your hopes are not completely fulfilled." Why couldn't we talk about that one? What does it take to really fulfill the heart? Is it children, or children just for a time, or because you think it's supposed to be that way, or to please your parents and your friends? Is it your work? Serving others, being religious, being a teacher, or a nurse? Can you be a business person serving others? Well, I know the answer to that is yes.

Our adoption time is coming closer, and now the nagging thought haunts me that maybe God never intended us to be parents; maybe we aren't supposed to adopt either. I've prayed to be led in a direction that would give purpose and meaning to my life. Going through artificial insemination was so emotionally hard on me. When you talked this weekend about the wonders of medicine and all they are doing now, all I could think was, "Yeah, they sure helped me, didn't they?" But then I wonder if I didn't let them help me enough. Maybe we should start artificial insemination again. Did we take things into our own hands, or did God lead us away from artificial insemination? You see how confused I am? I definitely do think too much. I can just hear you saying, "If she'd just relax and let whatever be . . . ," but that's not me, and that's not Dad either. We are so alike.

I remember once when you tried to talk about infertility, I was very cold and said we'd work it out ourselves. You see, I'm not blaming you for any mistakes; I've certainly made many. I guess we only find ourselves for fleeting moments in life—the hills and the valleys—oh, so many valleys, it seems.

I thought about how very close your neighbor and her daughter seemed to be and wished we could have that feeling again. I wondered how they maintained it after going through problems similar to ours. I was terrified the subject would come up in the evening conversation because I wasn't ready to handle it there when it had been avoided in our own home.

You said you "refrain from showing your real feelings for fear we might feel bound," but by not showing your real feelings, we feel only more "bound up" in our insecurities and loneliness. If I had been truly myself, I would have appeared overdramatic, selfish, unloving, and as if I wanted to be the center of attention. That's why Dad's sermon really hit home. I probably should have been truly myself. Christ would still have accepted me, weak and sinful as I am.

I know one prayer that has been fully answered in my life: that I would marry the right person. If I didn't have Craig as my strength and helpmate, I'd have been a "dead duck," and I mean that literally. I probably would have attempted suicide in the last year, but Craig is so good to me and so loving, I could never do anything to hurt him—I hope.

And I love you both so very much and only hope I will never behave so foolishly again. Instead I'll try to build our relationship by being honest and open. But I can't depend on myself alone. You see, I'll always need my parents.

Love,
Kaye

When I finished writing, I was thoroughly drained. Finally, it was out in the open. I was not the perfect daughter. I had been selfish, stubborn, proud, and I knew it; yet I believed my parents would understand and forgive me. I no longer had to keep up a front; I could be *me*.

When Craig came home from the office that evening, he could tell by my face and eyes that I'd been crying. After giving me a huge bear hug, he asked, "What's wrong?" Gratefully, I handed him the letter and asked him to tell me what he thought of it. He read it through, slowly, thoughtfully, and then suggested I wait a week before sending it, to see if I still felt the same way. That's what I did. I reread it occasionally, but my feelings didn't change.

I also talked to a close friend about whether to send it. She felt that children often have to teach their parents about life and feelings, stating, "Often after one is married, it's up to the child to teach parents how to stay close." That was all I needed to hear. If I hoped to reestablish our relationship, it was up to me. I mailed the letter.

Two days later they called, and we cried and talked for an hour. I felt very close to them for the first time in so long. I was warmed when they encouraged me to send them my manuscript. After we hung up, I knew our relationship had been strengthened by our openness and honesty. Even though it hurt at times, the results were well worth it.

Mom's next letter contained no small talk. It maintained the openness we established when they called:

Dear Kaye and Craig,

It was so good talking with you. I don't suppose anyone can really understand what anyone else goes through emotionally, although I believe most people do try. It's ironic that I've tried so hard not to interfere with your way of doing things because I felt you would make mistakes, like all of us, but you both had what it took to work things out yourselves. I've tried so hard to be a different kind of mother now that you're married, and it seems it was all wrong. So often I have tried to lead into things, but I couldn't pry.

We were concerned about your medicine and about the hospital. I didn't like to think you were there, but if you like your doctor, can I create doubts? I really felt I couldn't say anything. Once I was going to suggest something, I don't even remember what, and you said, "I know you are going to tell me to go to Dr. Jerry." Well, I wasn't, but I got your message —don't interfere. I still feel good seeing Dr. Jerry; it helps me. I have confidence in him, but I can't say that he is for you.

Kaye, why do you suppose I stayed longer with you than I did with Ruth and Jack when Kirsten was born? Not having a family certainly is not just physical; it is emotional and spiritual. Perhaps it isn't for you to have a family, although it's hard for us to imagine. We think it is for you, but we don't know all. We feel there couldn't be two better parents, but let us be confident that God, in his infinite wisdom, knows best. He knows what we want. He is able to do anything that we ask or think, so let's just leave it with him. This may sound like a pious platitude, but I've experienced just leaving it with him and a feeling of peace and rest. When we are in the valley, we have such a small view. Read Philippians 4; it helped me the other day. I'm also reading *To Live Again* by Catherine Marshall. The first part was helpful.

Love,
Mom and Dad

Less than a week later, Dad wrote:

Dear Kaye and Craig,

My first reaction is that it's good to ventilate and verbalize your feelings, just as you state. Whether by speaking or writing, it is most helpful to get the gut feelings out where you can look at them.

I regret that I was completely beat the week you came. You have no idea, Kaye, what inner tensions and burdens I was bearing. I hadn't slept a decent night the week before, and when we finally got to the lake, I was just dead. I remember your first night here, too; I could hardly keep awake and felt guilty. I don't blame you for feeling hurt, but there was nothing I could do. I'm not superhuman.

As for understanding and empathy, I guess I have failed miserably. We always loved your openness, and even though all teenagers are hard to manage, you were no harder than any other. Yes, Kaye, you are like me very much. I, too, am super-sensitive, and my skin is not very tough. You have so many talents that you should not feel depressed, although I must confess I also get fits of depression at times.

I'll be writing you more often. (Didn't know it meant that much to you!)

Much love,
Dad and Mom

Gradually I found ways to resolve my feelings about infertility, and my parents' letters and work on my book helped greatly. Luckily for me, the media was also beginning to push the concepts of career women and ecological care. Still, I became extremely angry when I read the feelings of one dissatisfied mother expressed in a letter to Ann Landers: "Parenthood is the most overrated job in the world. It's all pain and very little joy. . . . My husband and I have no one but ourselves to blame. No failed diaphragm, no missed Pill. We actually adopted our mistake after a long and happy marriage. The marriage is still hanging together (miraculously), but the 'mistake' is causing no end of misery. When one problem is solved, two others appear to take its place. Our advice to people thinking about parenthood is this: If your marriage is good—leave it alone. Don't take any chances on lousing it up."

"How cold, heartless, and ridiculous," I thought to myself. "Just because it's in print doesn't make it true." I became very aware of what the media was doing to me and began to select what was useful, ignoring what was painful. I also stopped comparing myself to others and began comparing my outward self to the person I really was inside. I set my own goals for happiness, finally rejecting the media's goals. After all, they were only trying to sell something. I wouldn't sell myself out.

And I was no longer bothered by what "the masses" think is right for a person of my age and marital status. I consciously ignored articles and commercials which made me feel inadequate, instead surrounding myself with opportunities for enjoyment, enrichment, and giving. Life is too short not to make the most of each day. As wise old Ben Franklin said, "Dost thou love life? Then do not squander time, for that is what life is made of."

I received another letter from my father shortly after his promise to write more often:

Dear Kaye and Craig:

The enclosed clipping [article on infertility] you may find interesting. We want you to know that, while we did not discuss the matter, that doesn't mean we aren't interested; it's just hard to know what to say.

I have never felt I could manipulate God's will through prayer to suit mine. I know of people who have been miraculously cured through prayer. But we should be willing to trust that God can say no to a prayer too. I must confess I haven't made this as much of a prayer petition as I should. I guess we have felt that, with your medical attention, the rest would follow in due time.

If you feel God is punishing you, that is not right. We have gone through that. Kaye, please don't for a moment think that we do not appreciate all you have done or that in any way we are disappointed in your not being able to raise a family. This has never entered our minds. We are grateful for your love, enthusiasm, and openness. We are so thankful for both you and Craig; we have said so many times that we think Craig is the greatest, and that you both seem to find fulfillment and happiness with each other. We couldn't wish for anything better.

I, too, get moments when I feel my life doesn't add up to all I would want. I think we all share at times a lack of fulfillment. So often I have seemed preoccupied with the parish when I should have spent more time with the family. Please forgive me if you feel we have neglected you. I promise to make this concern a daily prayer from now on.

If God wants you to have a family, you will. Then let us relax, in faith, believing it will come. O.K.? It's been good to spend these moments with you. *If you only knew how we love you.* Words even here seem so inadequate, but you know, I hope, that we feel you are living up to the highest ideals we could ever ask. Believe me.

All our love,
Dad and Mom

How I loved my parents and our regained closeness. They and Craig helped me become more open about infertility, more comfortable with it. One day when I met an old acquaintance she asked, "Do you have any children?" To my delight, it seemed like a simple, honest question, completely nonthreatening. And my answer, "No, we don't," had no hostility. I thought to myself, "Bravo, Kaye, you've come a long way, baby."

I began to search even harder for new experiences to enrich my life and found sharing with others to be greatly rewarding. At one choir rehearsal a member shared a poem by Helen Steiner Rice which deeply impressed me:

Not What You Want But What God Wills

Do you want WHAT YOU WANT when you want it . . .
Do you pray and expect a reply,
And when it's not instantly answered
Do you feel that God passed you by?
Well, prayers that are prayed in this manner
Are really not prayers at all
For you can't go to God in a hurry
And expect Him to answer your call . . .
For prayers are not meant for obtaining
What we selfishly wish to acquire,
For God in His wisdom refuses

The things that we wrongly desire . . .
And don't pray for freedom from trouble
Or ask that life's trials pass you by.
Instead, pray for strength and for courage
To meet life's "dark hours" and not cry
That God was not there when you called Him
And He turned a deaf ear to your prayer
And just when you needed Him most of all
He left you alone in despair . . .
WAKE UP! You are missing completely
The reason and purpose of prayer,
Which is really to keep us contented
That God holds us safe in His care. . . .
And God only answers our pleadings
When He knows that our wants fill a need
And whenever "OUR WILL" becomes "HIS WILL"
There is NO PRAYER THAT GOD DOES NOT HEED!

This friend and I discussed the correlation between the poem and 1 John 5:14, and I felt a close bond with her because I knew she had endured personal crisis when her daughter, a senior in high school, died of cancer. Yes, sharing is a true means of caring. I hoped to help others who were experiencing infertility by sharing my thoughts and emotions in my book.

One day the director of adoption at our agency asked me if I would participate on a panel titled "There Are No Children for Some" at the national convention of the North American Conference on Adoptable Children (NACAC). I enthusiastically accepted the invitation and worked diligently on my presentation. I could hardly wait for the convention.

When the big day finally arrived, I felt confident that

I could give rather than seek help, that I was ready to share what infertility had meant and did mean to me. I had never spoken publicly about infertility before, but the open atmosphere made me comfortable and confident.

One thing I talked about was the frustration of waiting for an adoptive child. The list below contrasts the wait of adoptive parents with the "normal" wait.

EARLY STAGES

Betty and Tom	Sally and Joe
Conceive and anticipate birth in nine months	Adopting in 18 to 84 months— or longer
• Betty and Tom find out they're expecting.	• Sally and Joe fill out forms, which takes two weeks.
• Betty and Tom announce to their family and some friends.	• Sally and Joe don't tell anyone; it's too far off.
• Betty experiences morning sickness and knows something is really happening.	• Sally and Joe are still taking temperature checks every morning and bringing sperm samples to a clinic.

MIDDLE STAGES

• Betty begins to "show"; now the world knows and smiles fondly on her.	• Some friends might know that Sally and Joe are planning to adopt, but seldom mention it.
• Tom is proud as friends acknowledge his virility.	• Friends begin to wonder why Sally and Joe don't have children.
• Tom and Betty shop leisurely, knowing in what season their baby will arrive. They start preparing the nursery.	• Sally sees some cute baby things, but can't buy them since it's still so far off.
• Betty gets a lot of attention and talks of her cravings and her discomforts.	• Sally and Joe seek out other adoptive parents to talk with. Sally becomes depressed and would gladly endure "discomforts" to have a child.

115

FINAL STAGES

- Betty and Tom take classes on childbirth and eagerly anticipate the birth of their child. Betty packs her suitcase.
- Betty delivers and friends come to visit with gifts and flowers.

- Sally and Joe go through more intensive counseling with their social worker and are "judged."

- The social worker visits the home to see if it is acceptable for a child.
- Sally and Joe wait, and wait, and wait, and wait.
- The social worker calls to say their child will arrive in three days. Sally and Joe frantically shop and prepare the nursery.

NEW PARENTS

- Betty is sore and extremely tired.
- The baby doesn't sleep through the night.

- Sally feels great!

- The baby sleeps soundly all night.
- Friends give showers.

The highlight of the convention was meeting Barbara Eck Menning, founder of Resolve, a newly formed organization which offers counseling, referral, and support groups to people with problems of infertility, and education and assistance to associated professionals. I was ecstatic to find that such an organization existed—after all the years I had bitterly complained that self-help groups existed for everyone except those who were infertile. I also met two other young women at this convention, both infertile and childless, and both eager to help others. We three agreed to start a Minnesota chapter of Resolve. We expended a great amount of

116

effort in forming and organizing this chapter and soon found ourselves on the speaking circuit throughout the Twin Cities area.

Things also began to move more swiftly in my work, and I was offered the management of a new studio, an exciting challenge I eagerly accepted.

I had a new lease on life. I loved my new work with interior design, I was close to my parents, and I was engrossed in my book. I had met new friends concerned about infertility and was becoming heavily involved in Resolve, an organization I felt a real need for. God did have a special plan for me; life did have purpose.

I no longer needed to desperately pursue some course to have a child. I was happy with our life, very happy. Craig and I would find other roads to give us fulfillment, to provide the joys of life we'd always had. Our adoption would eventually come through, and we would make that decision when it came. Yes—*make that decision.* By now we had waited almost six years, and I was beginning to think perhaps I was to be a career woman, that God had other plans for us which did not include a family.

Perhaps the wait was meant to bind Craig and me so closely together that we would never feel the heartache of the loss of each other's love. After what we had been through together, we felt overwhelming devotion for each other. I truly felt Craig was responsible for bringing me back to life again.

I was finding many rewards in life I would never have found if I had been a "normal" woman who married and within a few years became a mother. I was down a different course in life now, and who's to judge which road would have been better for me.

Life holds no sure answers to questions about whether to have children, how to proceed, how to conceive, how to deal with infertility, how to handle depression, how to keep mentally healthy. No universal guidelines exist. We must each find our own way, pursuing what we believe to be right. We can trust in the Lord, but we must also do our share. Oliver Cromwell said it well when he advised his soldiers: "Put your trust in God, my boys, but keep your powder dry."

I had put my trust in God. At last I was at peace. God had given me the inspiration and the strength to complete the overwhelming task of sharing our story. I did not have that kind of strength on my own. I had prayed long and hard that he would help me solve my problems. And he had. The book flowed from my heart.

"And this is the confidence which we have in him, that if we ask anything according to his will he hears us" (1 John 5:14).

Epilog

Craig and I finally were able to resolve our feelings about infertility. We looked positively at the childfree life and explored its possibilities for us. We looked at foster care as an opportunity to help others as well as ourselves. We looked at adoption as a special way of parenting. We explored career changes and other alternatives. I became more and more involved with my new career and had resolved infertility in my heart, mind, and soul. We were back to really living.

Then the call came. "Mrs. Halverson?" a cheery voice asked.

"Yes."

"This is Ms. Jones, your social worker."

"Who?" My mind searched for a connection with what I was hearing.

"Your social worker from the adoption agency. Are you ready to begin final processing for your child?"

After seven years of being on a list buried in a file

119

drawer, our name had surfaced. We might have a child in our home by Christmas. I was stunned. Only two months before we had been told we had possibly two more years to wait.

Ms. Jones explained that recently the waiting list had moved faster because many couples who were called had waited so long they were either committed to being childfree or had conceived children.

Now Craig and I had a choice. We could remain childfree, we could become parents immediately, or we could go through a nine-month waiting period before placement. We thanked God for hearing our prayers, and with joyous tears prayed for guidance.

By now I was actively involved in Resolve and was thankful to have friends with whom I could discuss my unexpected feelings of excitement, nervousness, and apprehension. Were we ready to undertake parenthood after 10 years of marriage?

"*Yes*," we said, "we would love a child in our home. The sooner the better."

Now a time of celebration could officially begin for us. Friends were called, showers were planned, and little packages and ornaments began to go on the Christmas tree with special love and tears—for a biological mother somewhere with a great amount of love and courage and for a newborn child. What a special Christmas this would be—a true celebration of birth.

But Christmas came and went. A New Year's Eve surprise shower, a special gesture of love, came and went. January, February, and March came and went. And the carefree Kaye of six months before hit another rock-bottom emotional low. The nursery door was closed, because it was too painful to look in at toys anxiously awaiting a little child. Our social worker had no answers; there simply was no child for us at this time. Were they changing their mind about us after our sessions with them to complete placement?

April and May came and went. My 10-year college reunion only proved to me how really *old* I was. Finally, the first week in June, our social worker called again, "You can come in on Monday and get to know your child."

Your child! *Our* child! A baby girl! Names we had discussed flashed through my mind. Sarah Marie? Anna Briana? Heidi Marie? That's it: Heidi Marie Halverson.

I hesitated to tell readers of the end of our childless life because many reading this book may have different options to resolve infertility. Infertility can be resolved in many ways, not necessarily through adoption. In fact, adopting can only be successful if infertility is resolved before placement. God had his hand in the timing of our becoming parents. He led us in special ways we never foresaw. How much pain we could have spared ourselves had we simply put our trust in him.

"Jesus immediately reached out his hand and caught him, saying to him, 'O man of little faith, why did you doubt?' " (Matt. 14:31).

Resources

Publications

The Boston Women's Health Book Collective. *Our Bodies, Ourselves.* 2nd ed. New York: Simon and Schuster, 1976.
Authoritative, easy-to-read text dealing with all aspects of female physiology, including infertility.

McNamara, Joan. *The Adoption Adviser.* New York: Hawthorn Books, Inc., 1975.
Contains information on the adoption scene, process, and alternatives, as well as a comprehensive directory of adoption resources available throughout the country.

Peck, Ellen. *The Baby Trap.* New York: Bernard Geis Associates, Inc., 1971.
An objective view of child*free* living.

Salkman, Victoria. *There Is a Child for You.* New York: Simon and Schuster.
Offers support and encouragement for adopting minority children.

Whelan, Elizabeth, M. *A Baby? . . . Maybe.* New York: Bobbs-Merrill Co., Inc., 1975. Presents reasons for and against having children.

Menning, Barbara Eck. *Infertility: A Guide for the Childless Couple.* Englewood Cliffs, N.J.: Prentice-Hall, Inc., 1977.

Presents reasons for male and female infertility and reports the latest advances in treatment, including embryo transplants and improved sperm bank facilities. Suggests how couples might take advantage of the alternatives open to them.

Organizations

Adoption Resource Exchange of North America (ARENA), 67 Irving Place, New York, NY 10003 (212) 254-7410.

Information clearinghouse on adoption in North America, especially finding homes for children with special needs.

AMEND, Dian Hoffman, 1548 Brenthaven, Floirisant, MO 63031.

Self-help group for parents grieving over imperfect or dead babies.

American Fertility Society, 1608 13th Avenue South, Suite 101, Birmingham, AL 35205 (205) 933-7222.

Provides information on medical specialists in infertility by geographic area.

Families for Children, Inc., 10 Bowling Green, Pointe Clare 720, Quebec, Canada.

Resource for international adoption.

National Organization for Nonparents (NON), 806 Reistertown Road, Baltimore, MD 20218.
Dedicated to promoting and supporting the decision to be childfree. (Founded by Ellen Peck.)

Organization for a United Response (OURS), 3148 Humboldt Avenue South, Minneapolis, MN 55408 (612) 827-5709.
Organization of adoptive parents. Prepares a bi-monthly newsletter containing adoption information.

Planned Parenthood Federation of America, 810 Seventh Avenue, New York, NY 10019.
Provides information about care, contraception, and doctors.

Resolve, Inc., P.O. Box 474, Belmont, MA 02178 (617) 484-2424.
National, nonprofit, charitable organization for infertile people. Provides free telephone counseling, referral to medical services or alternatives, support groups, public education, and printed material.

United Infertility, P.O. Box 23, Scarsdale, NY 10583.
Provides information on infertility.

World Family Adoptions, Ltd., 5048 Fairy Chasm Road, West Bend, WI 53095.
Resource for international adoption.

Patients' Bill of Rights

The information below may be of help to those who seek medical help in their struggle with infertility. It is from Barbara Eck Menning's *Infertility: A Guide for the Childless Couple,* © 1977, pp. 23-24, and is reprinted by permission of Prentice-Hall, Inc., Englewood Cliffs, New Jersey.

The following list of patient rights needs a brief explanation. A *right* is any situation that would be recognized as legal if the case were brought before a court of law. This list of rights is adapted from several sources, among them a model patients' bill of rights developed by George Annas for the American Civil Liberties Union. This list applies to hospitals and clinics and not to doctors in private practice. If rights are violated in private practice, the patient always has the recourse of seeking another physician.

Any patient, male or female, should expect the following from a concerned physician:

1. You have the right to be seen, fully clothed, in the doctor's office to discuss your case and ask questions *before* you are seen in the examination room. If this is your first visit to a doctor, you may request just an office visit and no examination, to see if you and the doctor are able to establish a good relationship.
2. You have the right to be seen on time or to be given an indication of the approximate wait you may have in case of emergency or unpredictable delays. Clinics can be especially negligent in this area. Your time is important, too!
3. You have the right to be treated respectfully, to be called by your proper name, and to have all interviewing and record-taking done in privacy.

125

4. You have the right to know exactly what each procedure will cost before it is done and what your insurance policy covers. You have a right to the highest degree of care available without regard to the source of payment.

5. You have the right to be talked to in language you clearly understand. If you speak another language, you have the right to have an interpreter present (a service available in most large hospital clinics).

6. You have the right to have everything explained to you *before* the doctor does it. He should explain the reason for the procedure, whether it will hurt, any possible side effects, and the results (or when the results will be known).

7. You have the right to know the name and dosage of any medication or solution given to you and the reason for any specimen taken from you and the results, when known.

8. You have the right to know your temperature, pulse, respiration rate, and blood pressure, and the interpretation of other physical findings that are made.

9. You have the right to be examined without a drape, if you wish, or draped in such a way that you can see what is happening. Some doctors have special mirrors and lights to allow you to see everything they do.

10. You have the right to be informed of any research studies to be performed on you and of any students of the health professions being assigned to you.

You may refuse either. If you accept, you have a right to full information about these activities.

11. You have the right to make your own decisions about your body. The doctor can only make recommendations. If you are unsure, get another opinion on your case before making important decisions.

12. You have the right to have all consent forms and documents fully explained to you before you sign them. You should never sign anything under pressure or duress.

13. You have the right to all the information contained in your medical record while in a health care facility and to examine the record on request.

14. You have the right to change doctors if necessary and to get satisfactory care and a respectful relationship. You should always be able to get a summary of your record forwarded to your new doctor at your written request. In order to effect change, you owe it to your previous doctor to tell him why you found him unsatisfactory.

It would be unfair to many fine doctors to imply that patients' rights are violated willfully or maliciously. Most doctors withhold information to spare a patient needless worry. They don't tell a patient something is going to hurt because they fear the patient will tense up or overreact. They don't tell a patient that a drug or treatment can have a certain side effect for fear of suggesting it. Some doctors truly believe that patients are comforted by a paternalistic relationship. Some use joking and familiarity to set the patient at ease. The doctor-patient relationship should be the same as any other service-consumer relationship. If you are dissatisfied, you should make your requests known. If the doctor is unable or unwilling to comply, you have the right to take your business elsewhere.

Communications are so important in the doctor-patient relationship that they deserve special emphasis. It is common for the patient to blame him/herself for not understanding medical terminology, abbreviations, parts of the anatomy, names of medication, and so forth. A person should try to become familiar with his or her body and its functions, but beyond that, it is the responsibility of the doctor or nurse to explain and interpret words to the level of the patient's understanding. The patient who is in a state of high anxiety or emotional stress hears and perceives *selectively* and may even have a partial or total memory lapse about things said in such a state. Therefore, the doctor should repeat important points several times and even ask the patient to repeat what he or she has heard. *What the doctor says is only half the communication. What the patient hears and understands is the other half.*